Nonnie Talks about Pregnancy and Birth: Volume Four of The Nonnie Series

Copyright ©2017 by Dr. Mary Jo Podgurski
All rights reserved

No part of this book may be reproduced in any manner whatsoever without written permission from the author. For information, write AcademyPress, 410 N. Main Street, Washington, PA 15301. The AcacemyPress is the publishing arm of the Academy for Adolescent Health, Inc.

The Academy for Adolescent Health, Inc. website is http://healthyteens.com/

Illustrations created by Alice Burroughs are the property of the Academy for Adolescent Health and are copyright protected. All rights reserved.

Photographs were purchased for use in this book or were donated and used with permission, for exclusive use in this book.

ISBN-13: 978-1543194326

Nonnie Talks about Pregnancy & Birth

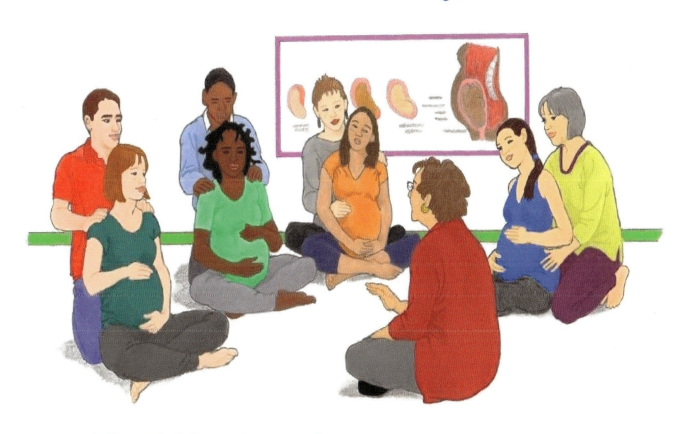

Suggested for children in grades 3 — 8 and their trusted adults

| An Interactive Book for Children and Adults | Written by Dr. Mary Jo Podgurski
Illustrations by Alice M. Burroughs | |

Dedications

For all the amazing people to whom I've taught
childbirth classes since the 70s
Thank you for sharing your lives
during such a treasured time.

With special gratitude to our reviewers:

Ann Grauer, AdvCD (DONA)
Anastasia Higginbotham, author of Ordinary Terrible Things
Barbara A Hotelling, MSN, BSN, LCCE, IBCLC, WHNP
Judith Lothian, PhD, RN, LCCE, FAAN
Sharon Muza, BS, LCCE, FACCE, CD(DONA), BDT(DONA)
Teri Shilling, AdvCD(DONA), LCCE, IBCLC
Tara Owens Shuler, M.Ed., LCCE, FACCE, CD(DONA),
Venus Standard, MSN, CNM, APRN, LMT, LCCE Certified Nurse Midwife
Bill Taverner, MA, CSE
Ngozi D. Tibbs MPH, LCCE, IBCLC
Allison Walsh IBCLC, LCCE, FACCE
Robin Elise Weiss, PhD, AdvCD(DONA), CLC, LCCE, FACCE

Special thanks to the wonderful parents
who generously shared pictures of their births:

Jazzmin Sims and Nicholas Foulks
Brandon and Janiya Williams

Introduction: Thoughts about a Child's Developmental Readiness for the Nonnie Series:

Many people ask me for help in determining a child's readiness for the books in the Nonnie Series.

Children today can glean information from online sources in a mouse click or smartphone search, but they are not always comfortable sharing their concerns with adults. Adults, conversely, may not know how to address complicated topics, or may think a child is 'too young' or unaware. I think the power of the Nonnie Series is the message "It's OK to talk about this together" – for adults and children!

Monitor your children's ability to process information. Maturity is often unrelated to reading ability; an adult can read and explain complicated words and concepts, but a child's curiosity and eagerness to embrace knowledge are important considerations. Adults need to 'articulate the obvious' when educating children. It's important to empower. Try paraphrasing this message: "I'd like to look at this book with you. I think you may be interested in the topic. We can read the book at your own pace. You can talk with me about anything, and I will respect you."

I suggest grade levels as opposed to age because I'm sensitive to reading ability, but I truly do not feel the books should be limited to one group. For example, not all 3rd or 4th graders will be developmentally ready for all the chapters in the books; the books should be read at a child's speed. On the other hand, not all 7th or 8th graders will be interested in interacting with an adult to address these topics, but some will enjoy learning and communicating with someone they trust.

No one is more important to a child than a trusted adult. Learning takes place when we process information; communicate with the young people in your lives and share your values with respect.

Each child is different. Let your children lead you. Their interest, more than their grade level or age, should be your guide.

Thank you for listening and caring about young people.

With respect and admiration,

Mary Jo Podgurski

Nonnie Talks about Pregnancy & Birth

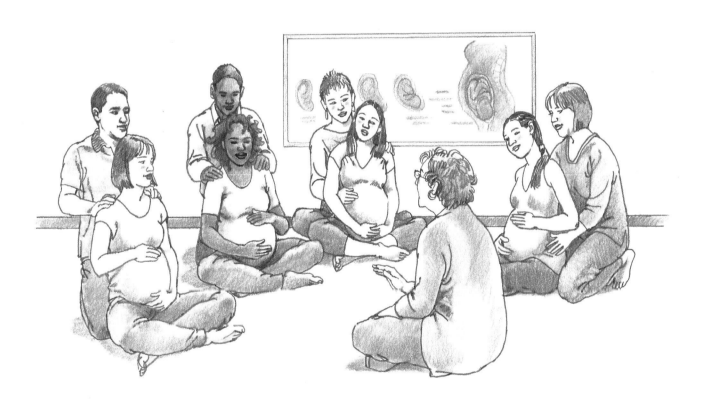

Suggested for children in grades
3 — 8 and their trusted adults

An Interactive Book for Children and Adults

Written by Dr. Mary Jo Podgurski
Illustrations by Alice M. Burroughs

HOW TO USE THIS BOOK:

Nonnie Talks about Pregnancy and Birth was created to be used by children and adults together. Please read this book with someone who matters to you.

For Children:
This picture means you may color the page if you wish.

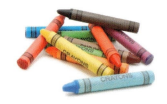

A red word means a word may be new. The Glossary on pages **79-83** will help with new words. Words written in blue are especially important messages or are for you, the reader.

A What do YOU think? page is a great page to help people talk with each other. Please talk with a trusted adult! Please listen!

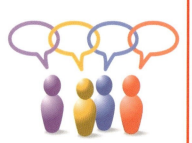

Most important:
Every person is different. Each child who picks up this book is different. Each adult who reads this book with a child is different.
Some ideas may be easy to understand. That's OK.
Some ideas may be difficult to understand. That's OK.

How to use this book:

For Parents, Teachers and Trusted Adults:

1. I strongly recommend reading the book without your child first. Consider any concerns you may have with the material and prepare for your child's possible questions.
2. The book is divided into chapters. The chapters are only suggestions; they divide the content to allow for pleasant learning. The book may be read as one part, two parts, three parts, four parts—it's up to you. You know your children best. Please monitor their attention, their interest, and their awareness and understanding of the concepts.
3. Chapters 4 and 6 contain complex topics. The reactions of my children's focus group were mixed - some 'got it' cognitively, while others became bored. You know your child. The chapters can be saved for later.
4. The topic of birth is life-affirming. Just as children's physical and emotional development are unique, so is their readiness for information. Please let the children you love be your guides.
5. The decision to include the topics of infertility and miscarriage was a careful one. My experience as an educator and a counselor tells me children hear more than adults realize. Their questions, in my opinion, require honest, respectful and empathic responses.
6. The language in the book is purposefully gender inclusive.
7. The What do YOU Think? pages should be completed at a child's pace, but are important. Learning takes place when we process information.

Most important:

Be aware of the "music" (tone of voice) behind your words. Adult modeling and acceptance of skills like respect and empathy as an ally are vital. **Please teach children the importance of respect.**

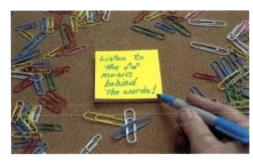

Nelson Mandela said: "No one is born hating another person because of the color of his skin, or his background, or his religion. People must learn to hate, and if they can learn to hate, they can be taught to love, for love comes more naturally to the human heart than its opposite."

Each Person is a Person of Worth. Please pass it on!

Mary Jo Podgurski

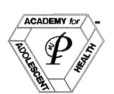

©2017, All Rights Reserved
Mary Jo Podgurski, RNC, EdD
Academy for Adolescent Health, Inc.
410 N. Main Street
Washington, PA 15301
1 (888) 301 2311
podmj@healthyteens.com
www.healthyteens.com

Chapter One: The Story Begins

Did you ever have a huge question?

Most children wonder about a lot of different things.

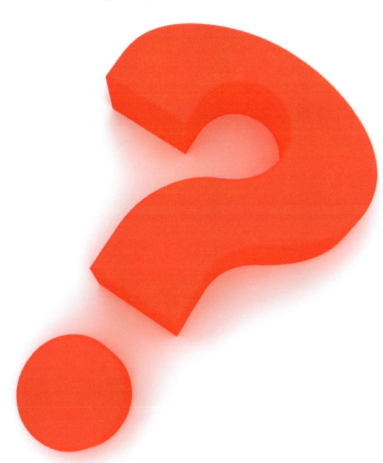

Would you like to read a story about two children with lots of questions? The story may answer some of your questions.

If you still have questions when the story is finished, please ask your parents or a trusted adult.

Once upon a time….

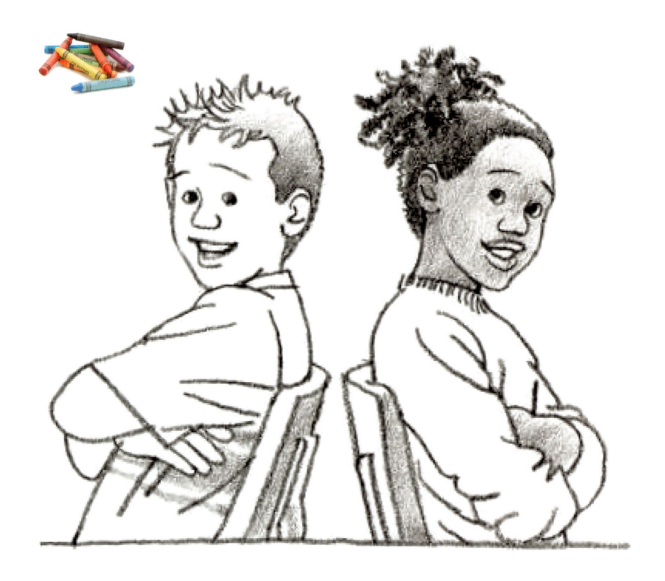

Alex and Tamika are best friends.

They can't remember a time when they weren't friends.

Their parents said they were even in the same play group when they were only two years old!

One day, Tamika and Alex were both so excited, they couldn't wait to see each other at school.

They texted each other right away.

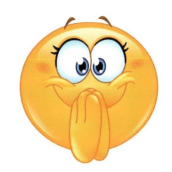

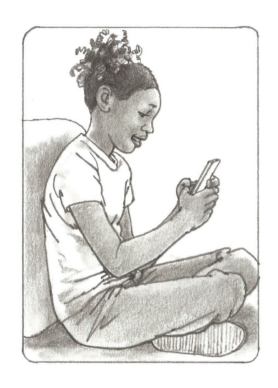

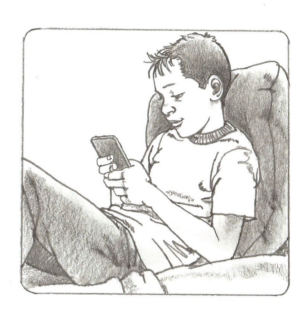

They were very happy.
They both had silly grins on their faces.

They wanted to share some important news about their families.
Their news was the best news ever!

 Can you imagine their surprise when they discovered their news was almost the same? Can you guess the children's news?

Chapter Two: Growing Families

Both the children's families are growing.
A *family tree* is one way to list all the people in a person's family. A family may not be the people to whom you are born. People may create families of people who love and support them.

Tamika's family is large.
Her family tree includes many people who love and support her.

Alex's family is also large.
His family tree also includes many people who love and support him.

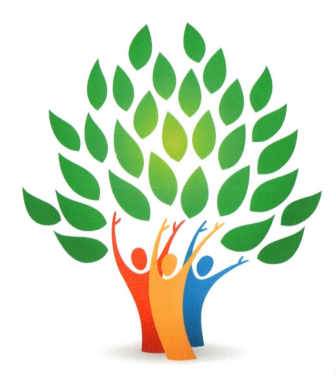

 Think about your family.

Do you have friends or trusted adults you think of as family?

Every person's family is different.

Your family is made of the people who love and support you.

Would you like to create your own family tree?

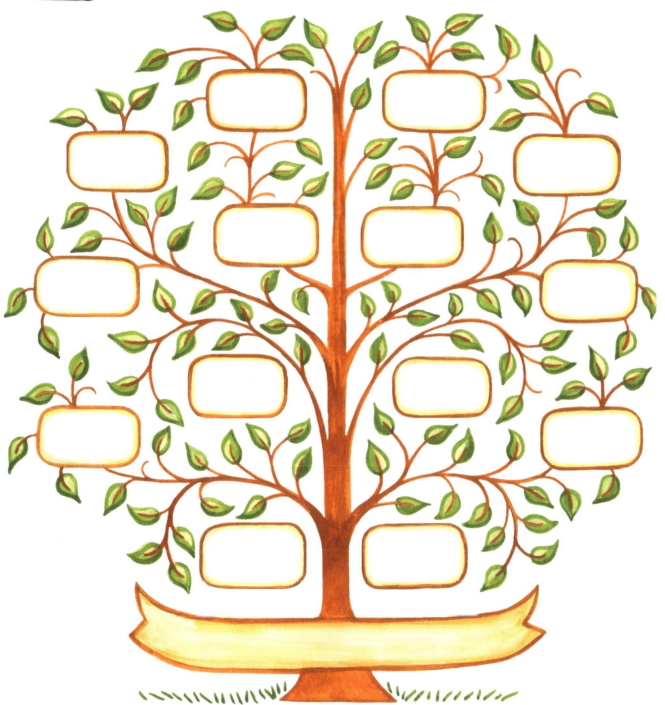

Tamika and Alex created their family trees when they were younger and Alex's Nonnie taught them about similarities and differences. Each family is different.

This is part of Tamika's family tree

Tamika's Mom's Side: Her mom's name is Nakisha and her grandparents are James and Monique.

Tamika's Dad's Side: Her dad's name is Louis and her grandparents are Emilea and Antoine.

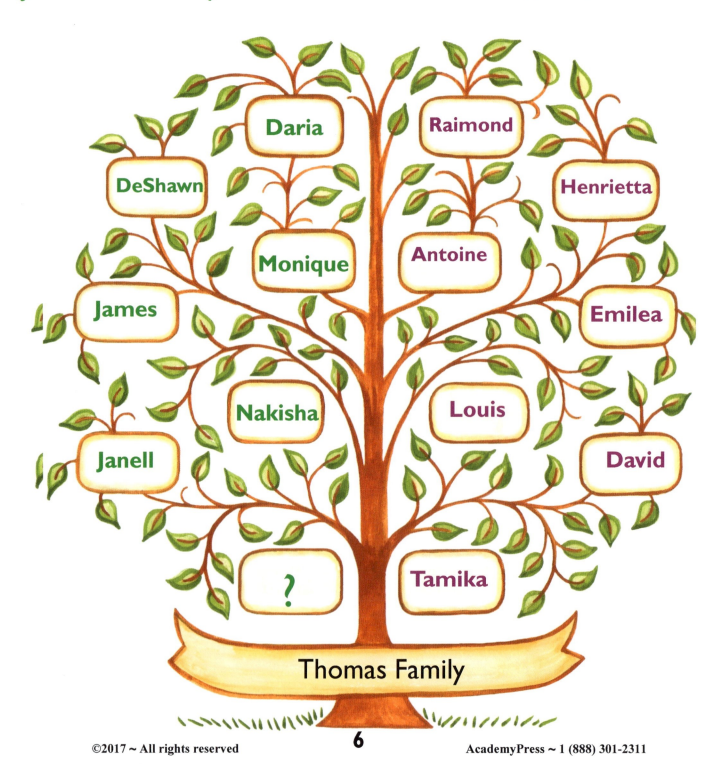

This is part of Alex's family tree

Alex's Mom's Side: His mom's name is Elizabeth and his grandparents are Tom and Sharon.

Alex's Dad's Side: His dad's name is Mike and his grandparents are Richard and Mary.

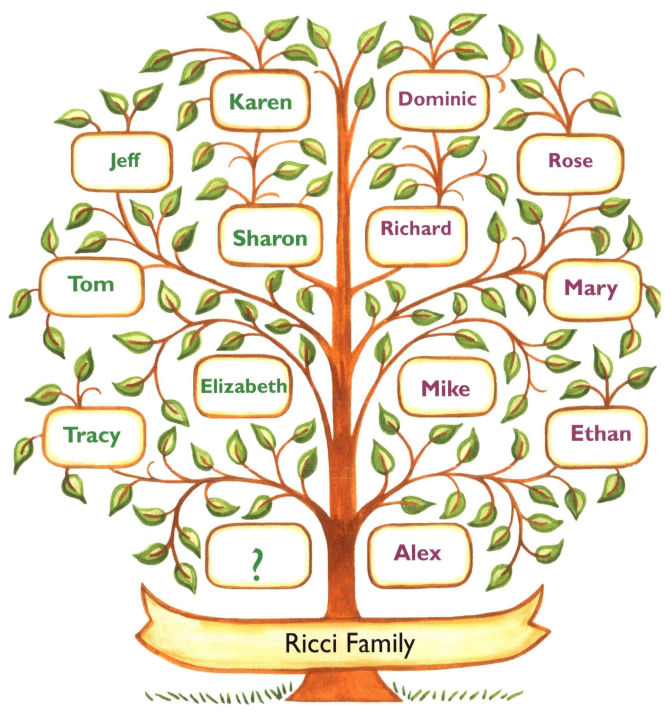

The children's news is about their families.

 Have you guessed? The children's family trees both include question marks. What do you think the question marks mean?

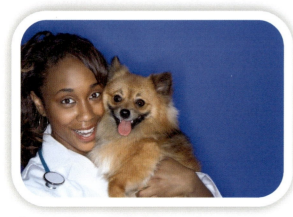

Both their families are growing!

Tamika's family includes her mother's younger sister, her Aunt Janell.

Janell is 29. Tamika loves visiting her. Aunt Janell is a veterinarian.

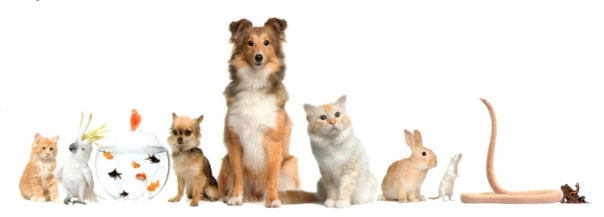

Her house is full of animals—two dogs, two cats, a cockatoo, a tiny orange parakeet, a rabbit, a spotted frog, a white rat, a bunch of fish, and a snake. Tamika especially likes the snake!

Guess what? Tamika's Aunt Janell is having a baby! Tamika will be a cousin!

Alex's mom's name is Elizabeth. Her friends call her Ellie. His mom is from a big family. She has 7 brothers and sisters, named Amy, Paul, Lisa, Evan, Nate, Erin, and Tracy.

Alex's parents are divorced. Alex lives with his step mom Teri and his half sister Alisha. He has a room of his own at his mom's house, too.

His mom's younger sister Tracy just turned thirty.

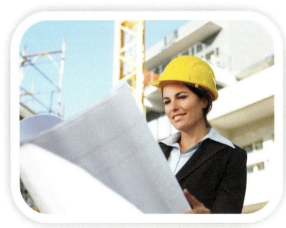

Tracy is an engineer, just like Alex's dad. Alex loves going to her office. He likes math and enjoys playing math games with her.

Her current job is working on the construction of a huge bridge over the river.

The river is near their city, and the children went to the construction site!

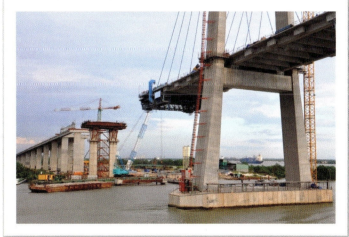

Guess what? Alex's Aunt Tracy is pregnant.

Alex will be a cousin, too!

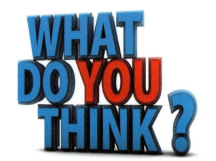

What do YOU Think?

New babies are fun.
Are there any new babies in your family?
Do you have any siblings?
Would you like to be a cousin?

Please draw or write your thoughts here:

Tamika and Alex know about babies.

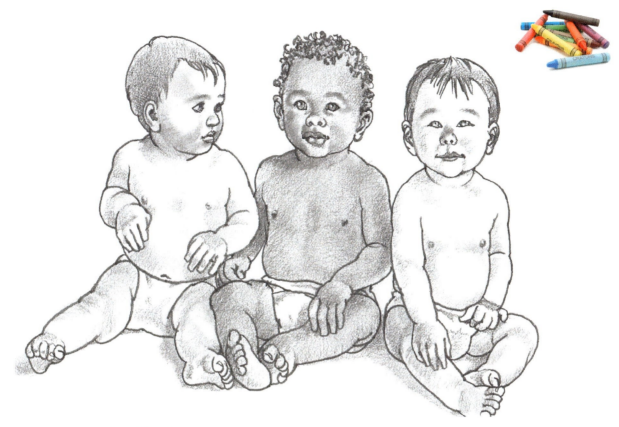

Alex loves his half-sister Alisha.

Her first word was 'Lex' - which is how she says 'Alex'.

Both children play with Alisha.

Alisha was the first baby in Tamika and Alex's lives.

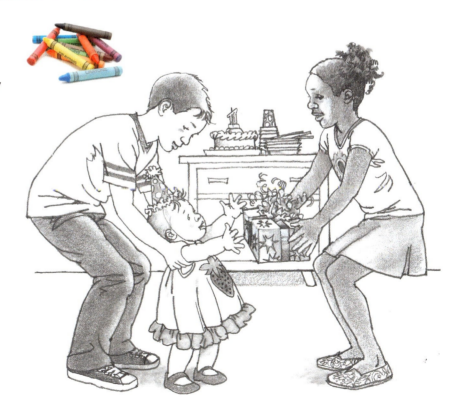

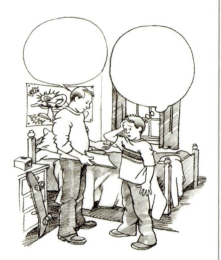

Tamika and Alex know about how babies start, too. When Alex's half-sister Alisha was born, they had lots of questions about where babies come from. They were younger.

Can you guess some of their questions?

The children's parents answered their questions, and Alex's Nonnie taught them. A Nonnie is a grandma.

Alex's Nonnie is a teacher and nurse. The children's parents often ask her to explain complicated things to them.

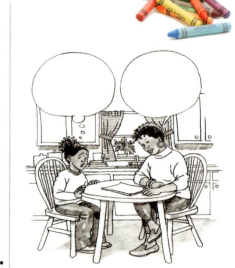

They love talking with Nonnie.

She respects them and listens to them.

She answers all their questions.

She always feeds them.

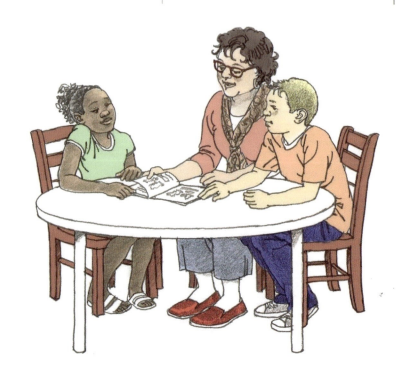

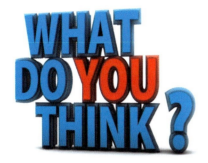

What do YOU Think?

Some adults think children are too young to learn about how babies are made*.

What do you think? If a child has questions, should those questions be answered?

Please draw or write your thoughts here:

*For more information about how babies are made, check out the book *Nonnie Talks about Puberty*.

Chapter Three: Pregnancy

Check out the way Tamika's Aunt Janell and Alex's Aunt Tracy look!

Their parents told them a pregnant person's abdomen grows during pregnancy. They were also told some people may say a baby is in a person's stomach, but it's not, and a pregnant person is not fat. Tamika whispered to Alex, "We're not little kids. We know this stuff." Alex agreed.

Their aunts look different to Tamika and Alex. The children were surprised to see their aunts' bodies. They overheard Alex's mom call Aunt Tracy's belly a "baby bump".

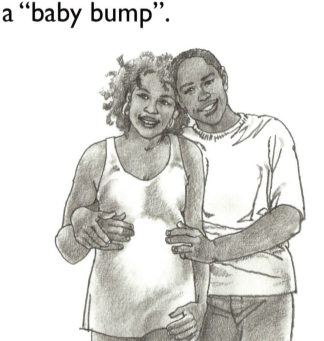 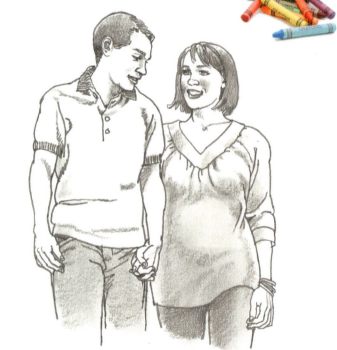

Tamika and Alex are very curious young people. Of course, they have questions about pregnancy and birth and babies.

Alex and Tamika's families were together, sharing a meal, when the children asked their questions.

Their parents' surprised reactions to their questions made both the children laugh. Their parents began to answer them, and then realized, like most children, they had some pretty detailed questions. Tamika and Alex asked:

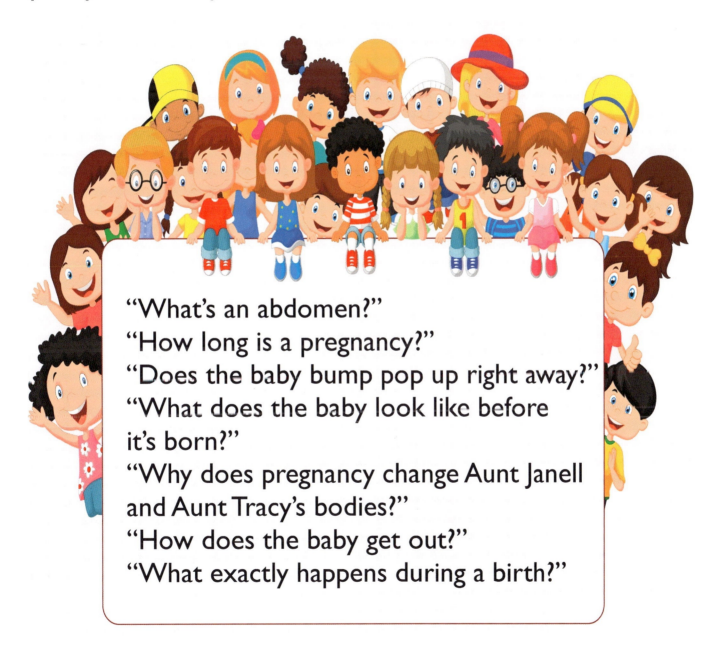

"What's an abdomen?"
"How long is a pregnancy?"
"Does the baby bump pop up right away?"
"What does the baby look like before it's born?"
"Why does pregnancy change Aunt Janell and Aunt Tracy's bodies?"
"How does the baby get out?"
"What exactly happens during a birth?"

Alex's dad Mike said, "We often ask Nonnie for help explaining things. This time, the topic of birth is one she really understands." The other parents agreed.

Mike continued, "I learned about childbirth from walking through my family room when I was growing up."

Tamika wrinkled her nose, "What?" she asked.

Alex's dad asked the children, "Did you remember Alex's Nonnie is my mom?"

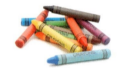

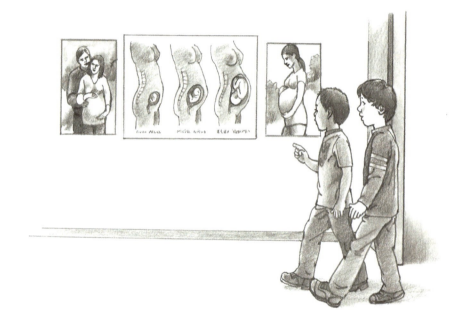

When the children nodded, Mike continued, "Nonnie taught childbirth classes in our home. One day I walked through her teaching room with my friend LeBron. There were posters everywhere. I told LeBron. 'Don't look around in my mom's room. You never know what you might see'."

Everyone laughed and smiled.

Tamika and Alex agreed. They'd like to ask Nonnie about birth.

When they arrived at Nonnie's house, she was just finishing teaching a childbirth class. The class is a special kind of childbirth class called a Lamaze® class. The children were very quiet. They slid onto their tummies on the floor and watched from the next room.

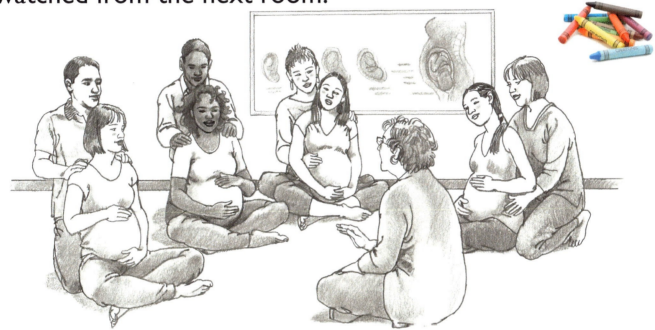

They heard Nonnie tell the people in her class she would see them next week. She told the class to remember their bodies know how to give birth. She played a game to help the birth partners know how to be supportive in labor.

When everyone left, Nonnie said, "I know you're there." Tamika and Alex laughed.

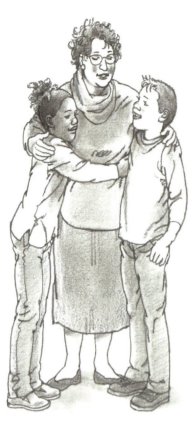

The children hugged Nonnie.

She said, "I hear you have some great questions. Shall we have a snack and talk?" They enjoyed apples and peanut butter. Nonnie likes to feed people!

She asked the children to write down their questions.

They wrote all the questions they asked their parents and a few more.

 Are you curious about pregnancy and childbirth? Please write your questions here:

_____
_____
_____
_____
_____
_____
_____
_____

Nonnie said, "We can talk about all your questions, and any thoughts you have as we talk." She asked, "Do you remember our guidelines—my promises to you when I answer questions?"

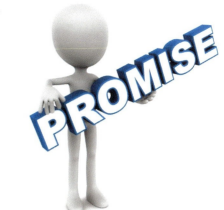

Alex and Tamika knew the guidelines very well. "Respect!" Tamika said. "We can even agree to disagree, but respectfully."

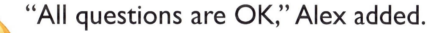

"All questions are OK," Alex added.

"It's OK to laugh," Tamika said, and gave Nonnie a big grin. "Because some things are just funny."

"As long as we don't laugh at others," Alex said, and Tamika said, "Yep."

Pleased, Nonnie asked, "Anything else?"

The children looked at each other and thought for a minute. Then, Alex said, "You'll tell us the truth, no matter what we ask."

"I will," said Nonnie. "Would you like to start with pregnancy?"

Chapter Four: Fertilization*

Alex said, "Yes, but first I have a big question. Bigger than all the others."

"Sure," Nonnie said. "Let's talk about it now."

"My mom told me Aunt Tracy and Uncle Ethan wanted a baby for a long time, but she never got pregnant." Alex said. "Last year, I heard them talking about going to a fertility specialist. They said Aunt Tracy and Uncle Ethan were experiencing infertility. What's infertility? And what's a fertility specialist?"

Before Nonnie could answer, Tamika said, "Well, whatever it is, it worked, because your Aunt Tracy is pregnant! I'm glad!"

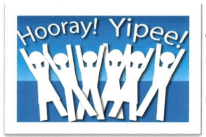

Alex agreed. "Yippee!" he said, looking at Nonnie. He knew his grandmother often said "yippee" when she was happy.

Nonnie agreed. "Let's talk about how babies are started. What do you remember from our conversations about puberty? What makes a baby?"

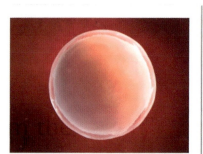

"An egg," said Tamika. "From the ovary."

*This chapter includes complex ideas. If it confuses you, you may read it later. Please enjoy this book at your own pace.

"And a sperm," added Alex.

"True." Nonnie said. "Another name for the egg is an ovum. Fertilization happens when the egg and sperm come together. How does fertilization typically happen?"

Tamika said, "Two people have sex. The kind of sex that makes babies."

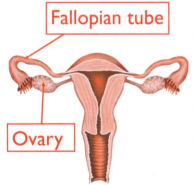

"Yes," Nonnie said. "The egg and sperm unite inside the fallopian tube. The fallopian tube is part of the female reproductive body parts. Reproduction means to…."

"Make or copy something else," said Tamika.

"I get it," Alex said suddenly. "Fertile has something to do with fertilization. Infertility means 'not fertile'."

Nonnie said, "Correct. A fertility specialist is a doctor who works with people like your Aunt Tracy and Uncle Ethan, who need help getting pregnant. Very few people need help."

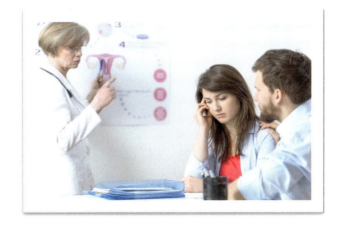

"How does the doctor help?" Alex was still curious. "How did the egg from my Aunt Tracy get fertilized by the sperm from my Uncle Ethan?"

"First," Nonnie said, "A doctor can help pregnancy begin by doing an IUI, which means sperm are placed directly into a uterus, so a pregnancy can start without sex. Hormones can be given. Typically, these kinds of procedures are enough to start fertilization."

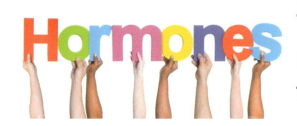

Tamika said, "I remember talking about hormones when we talked about puberty!" Nonnie was pleased.

Alex said, "My mom said Aunt Tracy had IVF. What's that?"

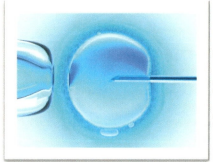

Nonnie answered. "The doctor removes eggs (ova—more than one ovum) from a person's ovary. The egg and sperm are united in the laboratory by a procedure called in vitro fertilization, or IVF. An embryo is created and transferred into a person's uterus."

"Most people's pregnancies start from one type of sex, though, right?" asked Tamika. Nonnie agreed. Tamika was correct.

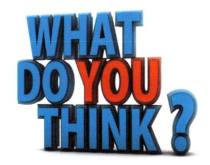

What do YOU Think?

Fertilization is pretty amazing, no matter how it happens.

Do you think it's amazing?
Have you heard of fertilization before?
Do you know anyone who went to a fertility specialist?

Please draw or write your thoughts here:

Chapter Five: Body Parts and Pregnancy

"Let's look at your questions. Your first question about abdomens is an easy one," Nonnie said. "I think you already know the answer."

Alex nudged Tamika, who smiled. "Yeah. We kind of asked that one just to see the looks on our parents' faces."

"Ah," said Nonnie, remembering these two young people were starting puberty. Puberty, she thought, can make a person a little testy. She asked, "Would you like to share?"

Alex said, "An abdomen is a person's belly," He touched his own abdomen lightly, "and a baby is not in a person's stomach, where digestion takes place."

Tamika agreed, but added, "Only a body with a uterus can be pregnant, though, right Nonnie? The baby grows in the uterus."

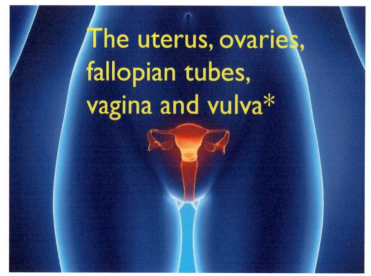

The uterus, ovaries, fallopian tubes, vagina and vulva*

*More information on the next page.

Nonnie was happy the children remembered their past conversations about bodies so well.

She asked, "Would you like to look at a picture?"

The children agreed, and she showed them this picture:

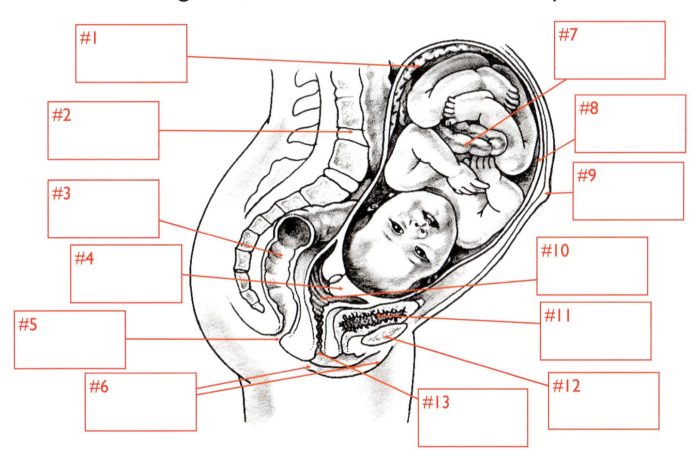

Nonnie said, "Let's play a game. Can you match the body parts on the picture?
You may use the names on the whiteboard."

   Can you match the names?

- Anus
- Belly Button
- Bladder
- Cervix
- Opening of Vagina
- Placenta
- Pubic Bone
- Rectum
- Spinal Column
- Umbilical Cord
- Uterus
- Vagina
- Vulva

Answers are on page 26

Tamika and Alex completed the diagram in a few minutes! They were able to guess some of the names, but the diagram gave them more ideas for questions!

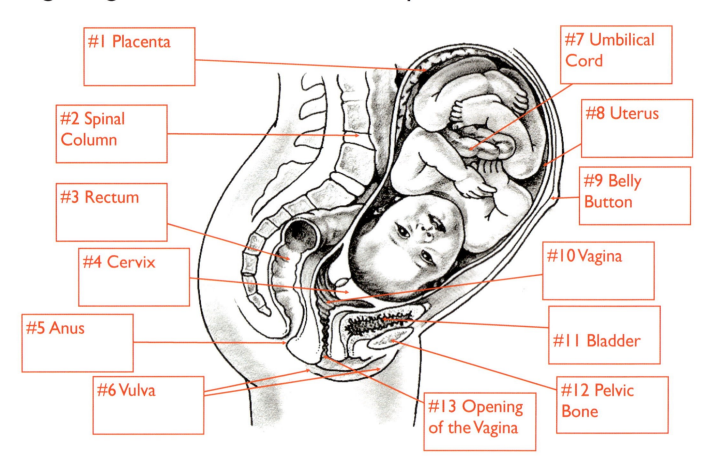

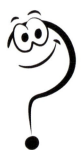

Nonnie asked, "What are your new questions?"

Tamika said, "I'd like to review some of the body stuff. I don't remember ever learning about a placenta?"

Alex added, "Yeah. Plus, why is the belly button an outie instead of an innie?"

Nonnie laughed. "As the abdomen grows, the belly button may change. Let's look at body stuff together."

"First, can one of you tell me what you know about learning the correct names for body parts?"

Both children answered quickly and confidently. Tamika said, "It's OK to talk about all our body parts. They belong to us."

Alex said, "Body parts are only dirty if we don't wash."

Nonnie agreed. She gave them a list of the body parts from the picture and their definitions.

> **#5 Anus:** The opening of the GI (gastrointestinal) tract through which solid waste (stool or poop) leaves the body.
>
> **#9 Belly Button:** The place on the body where the umbilical cord is attached in the uterus during pregnancy.
>
> **#11 Bladder:** The organ where urine is stored.
>
> **#4 Cervix:** The narrow, neck-like ending of the uterus—enters the vagina.
>
> **#1 Placenta:** Provides all nutrients and oxygen to the fetus.
>
> **#12 Pubic Bone:** Front bone of the pelvis (the bony cradle surrounding the abdominal organs).
>
> **#2 Spinal Column:** Part of the spine that supports the body.
>
> **#3 Rectum:** The final section of the large intestine ending in the anus.
>
> **#7 Umbilical Cord:** Connects the fetus to the placenta; delivers oxygen and nutrients to the fetus. Removes waste from the fetus.
>
> **#8 Uterus:** Also called the "womb" - the muscle that houses the fetus.
>
> **#13 Vaginal opening:** The opening to the vagina.
>
> **#10 Vagina:** Tube from the uterus to the outside of a person's body.
>
> **#6 Vulva:** The outside female body parts; the external genitals (genitals is a fancy name for those outside parts). Many people incorrectly use the term vagina for the vulva.

Chapter Six: Development!*

The children matched the body parts again. They made sense to them.

"Are you curious about anything?" Nonnie asked.

Alex pointed to the picture. "What's a fetus?"

Nonnie opened one of her books. This book was about pregnancy. She showed the children a picture of intrauterine development (the growth from fertilization to baby that happens inside a uterus during pregnancy).

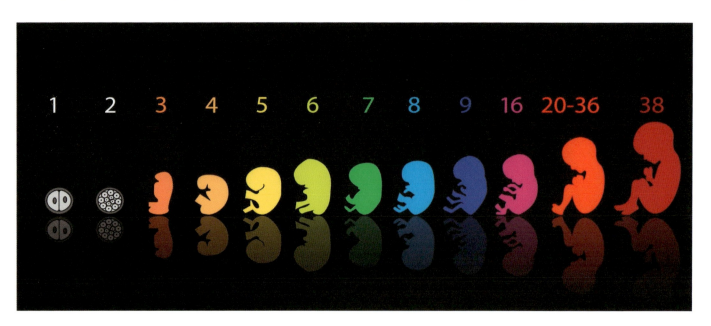

"Wow!" Tamika said.

Alex said, "We go through a lot of stages before birth?"

*This chapter includes complex ideas. If it confuses you, you may read it later. Please enjoy this book at your own pace.

Nonnie said, "Ever since the first biology class during my nursing training, I've been fascinated by pregnancy. There are some very unusual words in this part of the story. Are you interested?"

Tamika snorted. "You know us, Nonnie!" she said.

"I do," Nonnie said. "After fertilization, the egg and sperm become a zygote. The next phase of development is the blastocyst, which implants (sticks) in the wall of the uterus. The blastocyst is then called an embryo. At 8 weeks, the embryo is called a fetus."

Very Early Pregnancy

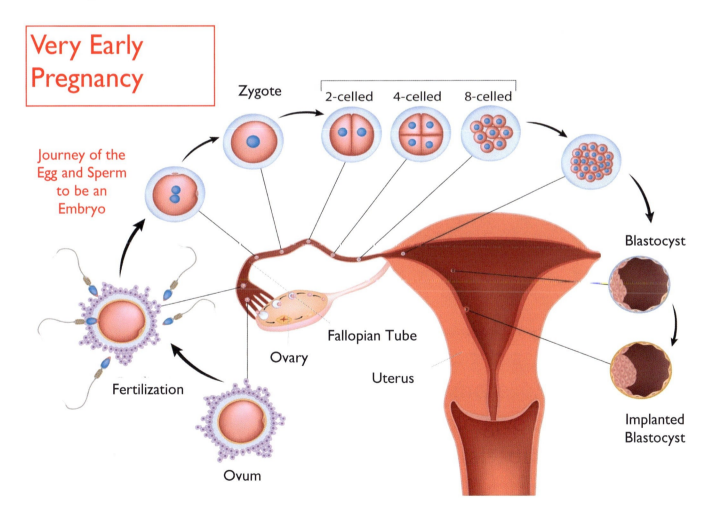

Both children looked a little overwhelmed. Nonnie said, "This development is very quick, but the embryo is so small. At four weeks, an embryo is the size of a poppy seed, at seven weeks, the size of a blueberry, and at eight weeks, the size of a kidney bean."

Tamika said, "Wow! What about our aunts' babies?" Alex pulled a picture up on his phone. "This is a picture of my Aunt Tracy's baby right now," he said. "What does 2nd trimester mean?"

Tamika laughed. "I have Aunt Janell's picture and it looks like yours! My aunt said it's called an ultrasound picture."

Nonnie said, "When I was pregnant, we didn't have ultrasound pictures. Can you see the face?"

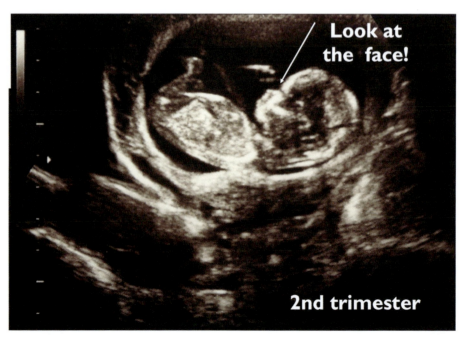

When the children saw the outline of the face, Nonnie answered Alex's question. "One of your first questions was, How long is a pregnancy? A pregnancy lasts an average of 37—42 weeks, and is divided into trimesters.

The first trimester lasts from Week 1—12
The second trimester lasts from Week 13—28.
The third trimester lasts from Week 29—42."

"Wait a minute," Alex interrupted. "Are you saying my Aunt Tracy is already in her 2nd trimester and I just found out about her pregnancy?"

"Yeah," Tamika looked angry. "My Aunt Janell is in her 2nd trimester, too. No one told me."

Nonnie smiled, but the children thought her smile looked sad. "You sound annoyed," she said. "Your families wanted to wait for the pregnancies to reach the 2nd trimester because they wanted to protect you. Not all pregnancies are OK. A miscarriage can happen when a pregnancy ends early. This can be a very sad time. A miscarriage is no one's fault."

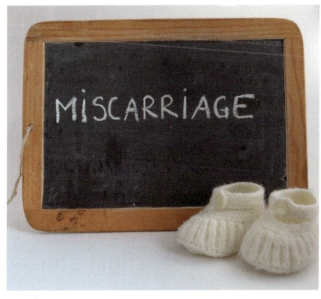

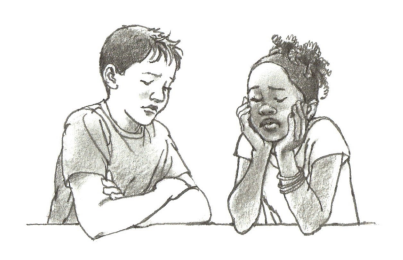

The children were quiet, and then they talked to each other in soft voices. Nonnie waited while they thought about what a miscarriage might mean.

Finally, Alex said, "We understand. It would be very sad to have a dream like a pregnancy end. We're glad our aunts' pregnancies are going well."

Tamika added, "Why do adults think kids can't handle sad things? We know it's OK to cry and be sad."

Nonnie disagreed, with respect. "This is my opinion," she said. "I think many adults do believe children are able to deal with sad things. I know your parents respect you both and treat you like young people, not little kids. Can you think of other reasons adults might protect children?"

"So we're not sad," Tamika guessed. "Maybe, so we're not afraid."
Alex said, "So we are happy."

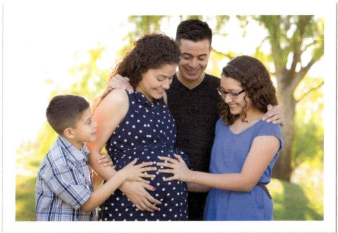

Nonnie said, "I'm very proud of the way you think about others. Shall we move on?"

The children were ready to learn about what was happening inside their aunts' bodies. "You can see a pregnant person's body change on the outside," she said. "Feeling a baby kick is amazing!"

"I felt the baby kick!" crowed Tamika. "Me too," Alex grinned. "So weird, but so great."

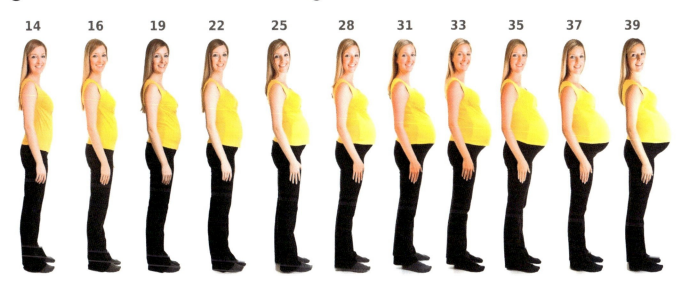

"Each person is different," Nonnie said. "Each pregnancy is different, too."

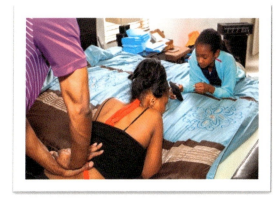

"I've attended a lot of births," Nonnie continued. "Each birth is different as well."

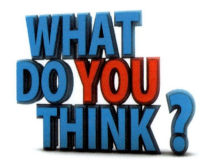

What do YOU Think?

Tamika and Alex think adults try to protect children from sad things.

Do you think adults in your life protect you from hearing about sad things? How do you feel when you think about the idea of a miscarriage?

Please draw or write your thoughts here:

"What happens inside the uterus, Nonnie?" Alex asked.

Nonnie asked, "Do you remember anything about the uterus?"

"It's a very strong muscle," Alex said. "The kind of muscle a person doesn't control. What's the name for that kind of muscle, Nonnie?"

"An involuntary muscle, Alex," Nonnie said. "Very good."

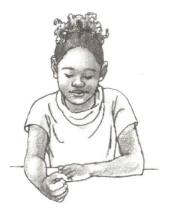

"The uterus is small before a pregnancy," Tamika made a fist. "Like my fist. It gets big, like a watermelon, at the end of a pregnancy."

A uterus

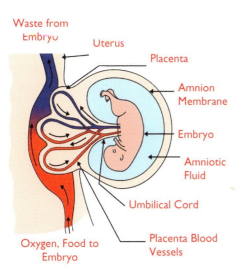

"Excellent, Tamika," Nonnie said. "The uterus is perfect! The placenta keeps the fetus alive by providing nutrients and oxygen through the umbilical cord. Amniotic fluid (a special liquid) surrounds and protects the embryo."

"Whoa," Alex said, "Weird!"

Chapter Seven: Inside the Uterus

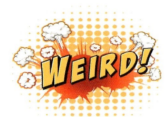

Nonnie laughed. "I guess weird is an OK word, Alex."

"A good weird," Alex added, smiling.

"Can you show us pictures of what's happening inside the uterus?" Tamika asked.

"Absolutely." Nonnie booted up her laptop. "Check it out."

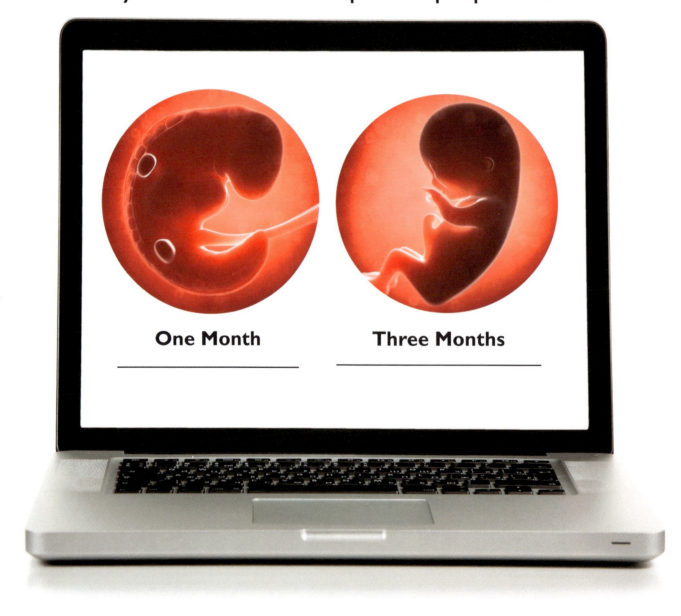

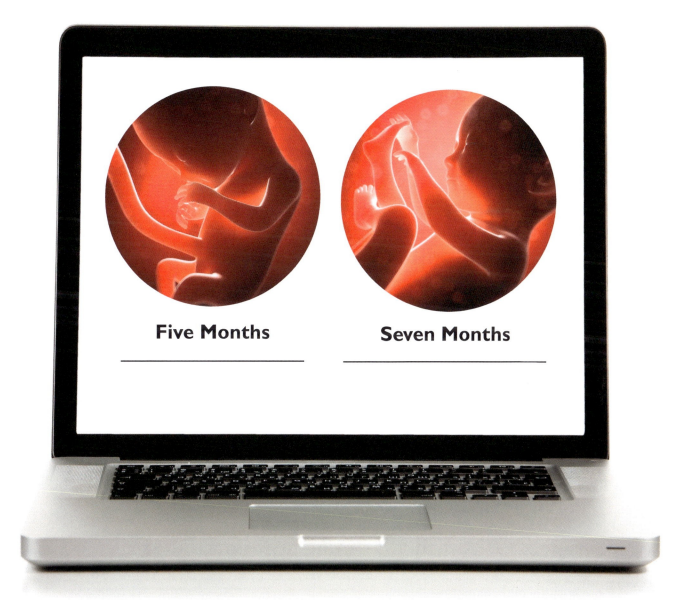

Five Months   Seven Months

"I love this," Tamika was excited. "Maybe I'll study biology when I'm older."

Alex grinned at her, "I thought you were going to be a singer."

"I don't know." she said. "Maybe I'll study biology, too."

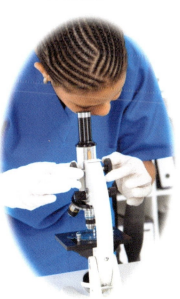

"I'll bet the baby takes up a lot of room inside!" Alex suddenly realized something. "I don't have a uterus, Nonnie, so I won't be pregnant."

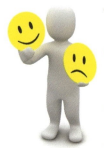

"True, Alex." Nonnie was curious. "Are you happy or sad?"

"Both, honestly," said Alex after thinking. "The pregnancy thing is kind of scary, but amazing, too."

Both Nonnie and Tamika agreed. "Just because I have a uterus, Alex, doesn't mean I'll ever be pregnant." Tamika said. "Right, Nonnie?"

"Correct." Nonnie smiled. "Having a baby is an adult choice. You have time to decide." She showed the children her posters. "Watch how the abdomen changes."

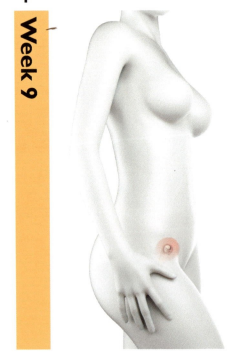
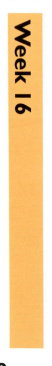
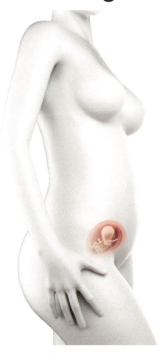

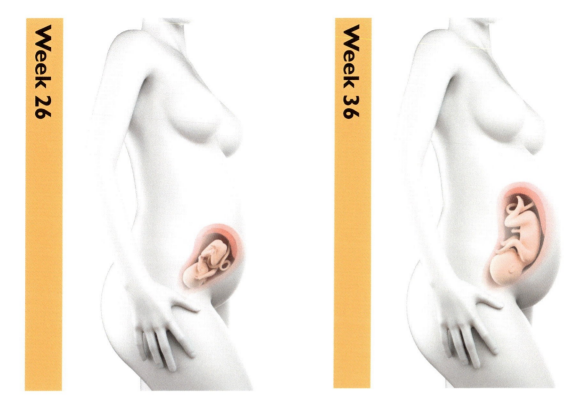

Tamika started giggling. Nonnie and Alex looked at her, curious.

"What's up, Tamika?" Alex wanted to laugh, too.

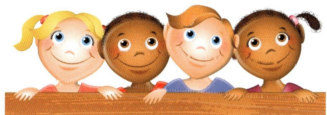

"Where are the people's heads and legs?" Tamika asked. "Heads are important."

"Feet and legs are, too," Alex added, grinning.

Nonnie didn't laugh. "You're correct, honey. Too often, posters and pictures of pregnancy show headless people. I asked my artist friend Alice to draw some pictures of full bodies. Let's look at those pictures."

"Would you like to color these pregnancy pictures?" Nonnie asked. The children said, "Yes."
Tamika laughed again. "These pictures are better, Nonnie, but I still don't see legs!"
The drawings start with the third month.

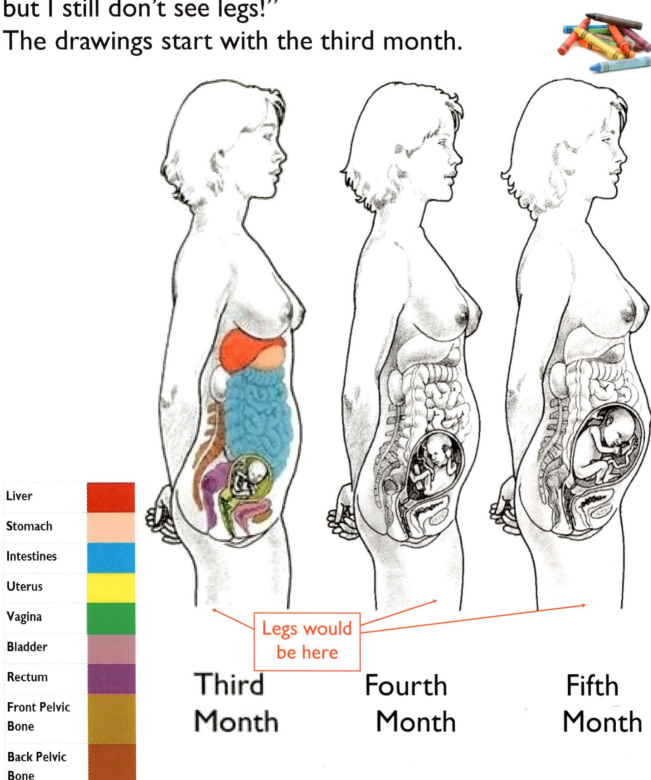

Liver
Stomach
Intestines
Uterus
Vagina
Bladder
Rectum
Front Pelvic Bone
Back Pelvic Bone

Legs would be here

Third Month   Fourth Month   Fifth Month

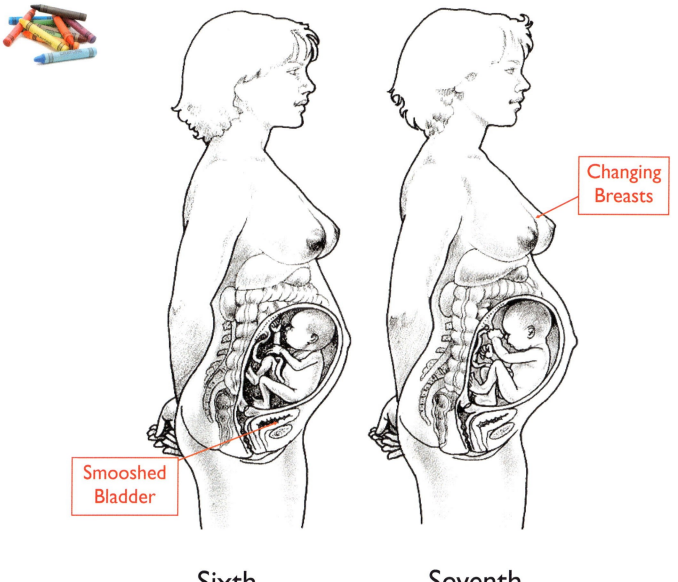

Sixth Month   Seventh Month

"What do you notice in the pictures?" Nonnie asked.

"The breasts get bigger," Alex said. "The breasts make milk for the baby."

"The bladder is all smooshed," Tamika noticed. "I guess pregnancy means knowing how to find bathrooms!"

"All the other body stuff gets squished, too," Tamika said. "The stomach gets pushed up."

"The belly button is an outie here, too," said Alex.

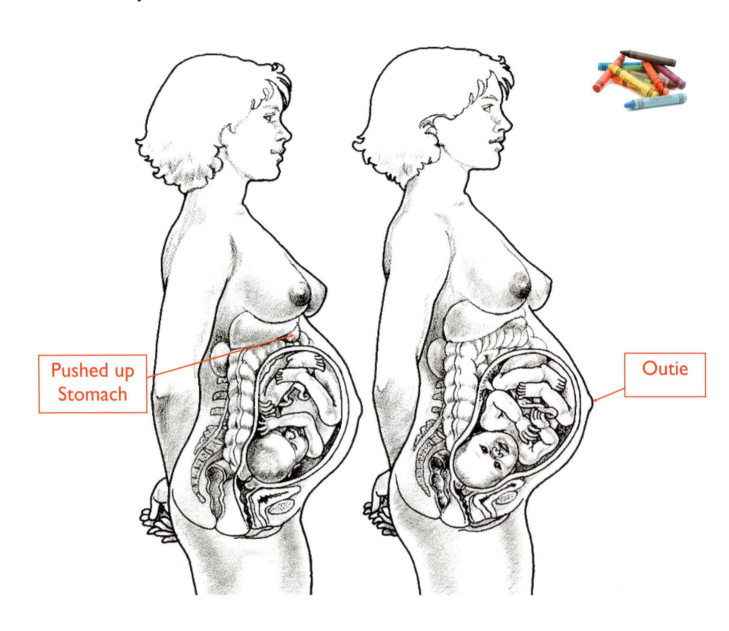

Eighth Month

Ninth Month

Chapter Eight: Pregnancy Feelings

"What does a pregnancy feel like, Nonnie?" Tamika asked, still looking at the pictures. "The body really changes."

"Great question, Tamika," Nonnie smiled. "I loved being pregnant, but not everyone enjoys the feelings of pregnancy."

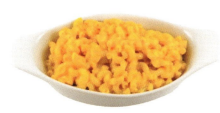

"I heard my mom say Aunt Tracy craved mac n cheese. What's a craving?" Alex asked.

Tamika laughed, "Wanting pickles, right?"

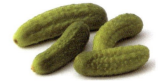

"A craving is when a person wants something special to eat. Some people may crave pickles or ice cream during pregnancy, but every person is different. Some people don't crave any special food." She thought for a moment, then grinned. "I wanted acorn squash."

"Ewww," said Tamika. "Yum," said Alex. The children looked at each other, and Alex said, "Nonnie, we're not pregnant, but we're craving a food."

"Nachos," said Tamika. Nonnie laughed. They made nachos together and had a second snack.

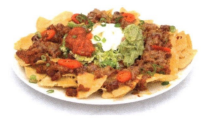

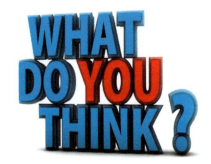

What do YOU Think?

A craving for a special food during pregnancy may be a myth.
A myth is probably not true.

Do you ever crave any special foods?
Have you heard any myths about pregnancy?

Please draw or write your thoughts here:

Nonnie was curious. She asked, "The idea of craving pickles and ice cream during pregnancy is a common myth. Do you know any other myths about pregnancy?"

Alex said, "I heard my stepmom tell Aunt Tracy it wasn't safe to dye her hair during pregnancy." Nonnie nodded. "Dyeing hair is OK. Another myth."

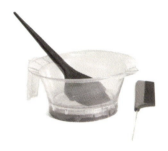

Tamika said, "I heard lifting their arms above pregnant people's heads will hurt babies."

"A common myth," said Nonnie. "This myth comes from a fear of the umbilical cord going around the baby's neck. There's no connection between the cord and the pregnant person's arms. Exercise during pregnancy is good."

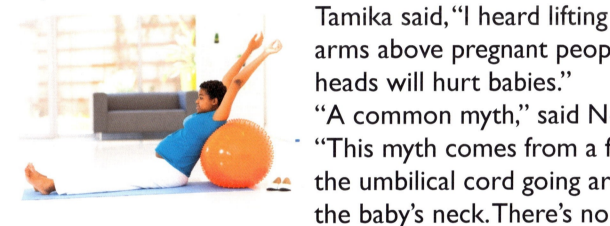

"What about cats?" Alex said. "Uncle Ethan said he takes care of the cat litter box now. Is it OK if Aunt Tracy pets Pepper?"

"Yes, she can pet a cat," Nonnie said. "Toxoplasmosis is an infection caused by a parasite carried by cats. As long as the pregnant person doesn't clean the litter box, all should be OK."

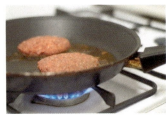

"Aunt Janell said she felt sick if she smelled certain foods, like hamburger cooking." Tamika said.

"Yes," Nonnie agreed. "Nausea is pretty common during pregnancy, and odors might increase the feeling."

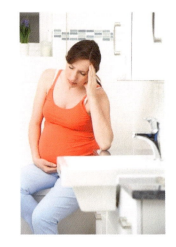

"Do people throw up? I hate throwing up." Alex looked ill just thinking about it.

"Sometimes." Nonnie said.

"What else happens during pregnancy?" Tamika asked.

"In early pregnancy, a person may be very tired, even if no one can see a change in the person's body. At the end of a pregnancy, the baby takes up a lot of room, like in the pictures.

Many people experience backache and need to use the rest room a lot."

"Aunt Janel has a huge body pillow." Tamika said. "She said it's tough to get comfy at night."

"Yes," Nonnie said. "Pregnancy causes many changes.

Emotions or feelings can change during pregnancy, too."

"Like in puberty," said Alex. "Do hormones make a pregnant person moody?"

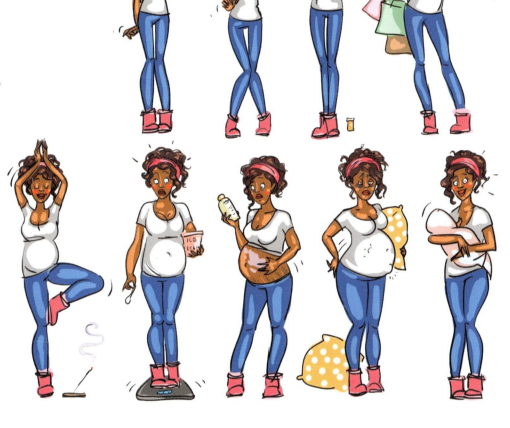

"Maybe," Nonnie said. "Think about it. A pregnancy can last a long time—up to 42 weeks. A person may be concerned about labor and birth. Becoming a parent is a big deal, too. Being excited is normal, but so is feeling worried or even afraid.

I like teaching childbirth classes. Preparing for birth can ease pregnancy fears and support parents' feelings."

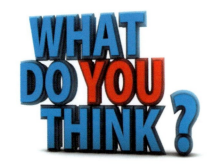

What do YOU Think?

Bodies change during pregnancy.

Are you surprised by the changes?
What feelings are new to you?
Which body changes do you think would be "weird"?
Would you use Alex's word "weird" to describe them?

Please draw or write your thoughts here:

Tamika started giggling again.

Alex started to laugh, too, because laughing can be contagious.

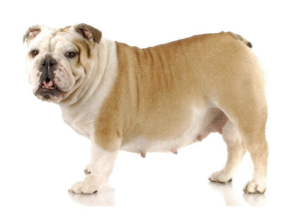

Tamika explained. "I just thought about your dog, Mitzie, Alex. Remember when she had her puppies? I never thought about pregnancy, or realized Mitzie was having puppies. I just loved playing with them!"

"You were younger, Tamika," Nonnie said gently. "You didn't understand."

"I like understanding," Tamika said proudly.

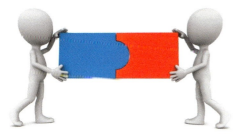

"Me too," said Alex. "Learning is like figuring out a puzzle. When you put the pieces together, you 'get it'. Things make sense."

Tamika and Alex are correct. When things make sense to you, the puzzle of learning is complete.

Are there any animals in your life? Have any of them given birth? If so, list their names here:

"Wait a minute," Tamika's mouth was open in a wide O. "I never got it until now...belly buttons…" She turned to Alex, her voice kind of high and excited. "I just realized. Belly buttons."

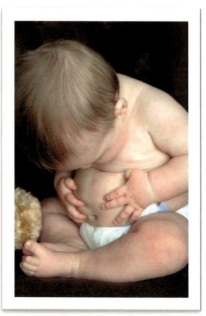

Alex shook his head. "What about belly buttons?"

"Our belly buttons are where we were attached to our moms by an umbilical cord." Tamika declared. "Before we were born. Did you know?"

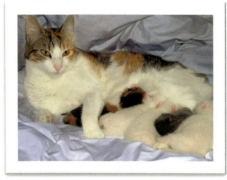

Alex remembered. "I honestly didn't think about it, but I was with Pepper when her kittens were born. I guess I never connected the kittens' umbilical cords with people!"

The children were so excited. Alex said, "I think we need pizza, Nonnie. My brain needs food." Nonnie smiled. Nachos weren't enough.

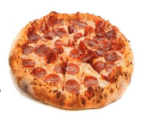

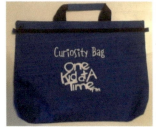

Nonnie called their favorite pizza place. While they waited, the children colored and talked about their aunts. They wrote more questions for Nonnie's Curiosity Bag.

Alex said, "My Uncle Ethan is so happy about the baby, too. We haven't talked about him."

"You're right," Tamika agreed. "Or about my Uncle David."

Nonnie said, "We were focused on pregnancy. You're correct. Partners in birth are really important. Did you notice my class earlier?

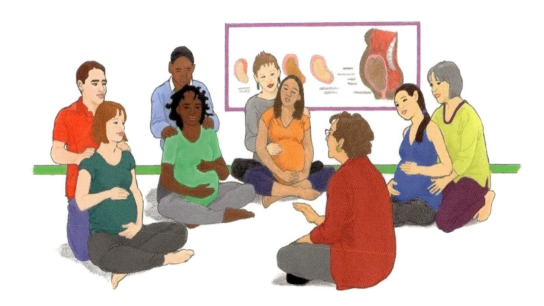

Two of the partners are dads. One partner group is of two women who are life partners as well as birth partners. One partner is a grandma. A birth partner gives support during labor and birth. Being a birth partner is wonderful."

Alex was curious about Nonnie. "Was Pop-op your birth partner when my dad was born?" Nonnie smiled and said, "Yes. He was with me for all three of my births."

Chapter Nine: Childbirth

"Do you have any new questions about birth?" she asked. The children emptied the Curiosity Bag. Along with their first questions: "How does the baby get out?" and "What exactly happens during a birth?" were four new questions:

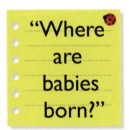 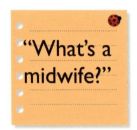 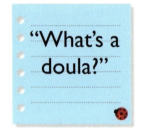 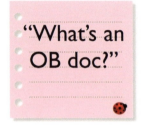

"Great questions," Nonnie said. "I'd love to know why you asked them."

Tamika said, "I heard my Aunt Janell talk about having a home birth. I thought babies were born in hospitals."

"Not always," Alex said, "My baby sister was born at home."

"You're right, Alex," Nonnie said. "Alisha was born at home. I was there. Many people give birth in hospitals, others at home."

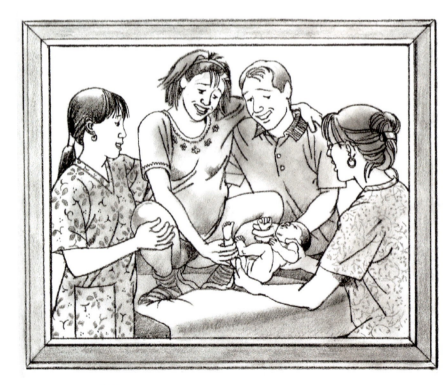

Then Alex said, "My Aunt Tracy says she is going to a midwife. I've never heard of a midwife."

"My Aunt Janell talked about using a doula." Tamika said. "We overheard our parents talking about an OB doc."

Nonnie said, "Each time I talk with you, I learn more about you. You're very good listeners. You're also good at eaves-dropping."

Alex laughed. "We learn stuff by listening, right, Tamika?"

"We're like your dog, Bravo, Nonnie." Tamika seemed excited. She was fidgeting on her chair. "He always looks like he's listening to us."

Nonnie laughed. "Bravo does look like he's always listening. Maybe he is, or maybe it's the size of his ears! I love the way you two ask questions. What if we start by talking about your first two questions? Answering what happens during a birth and how a baby gets out of the uterus will help us talk about your new questions. OK?"

Tamika rubbed her hands together. "Finally. Yes. How does the baby get out?!"

Alex said, "I hope you have pictures, Nonnie. I learn best when I see things."

"I have lots of pictures, Alex." Nonnie opened a huge scrapbook. "First, let's talk about how babies are born. I also want to share some pictures of doulas and midwives and OB docs."

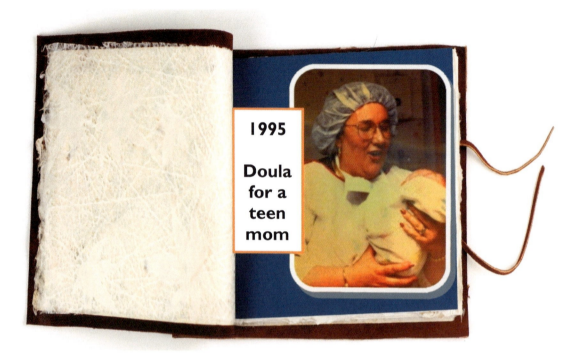

"Oh my goodness," Tamika said. "Is that you, Nonnie."

"It's me a long time ago," Nonnie laughed.

Alex said, "We have pictures at our house of you when you were younger. You kind of look the same."

Nonnie laughed. "Not really, Alex, but what a sweet thing to say."

She continued, "The first thing you need to know about giving birth deals with choices. People have options during pregnancy.

1. They can pick an OB or family practice doctor or a midwife for care.
2. They can select a childbirth class and learn about their bodies and the normalcy and reality of giving birth.
3. They can decide to take a prenatal exercise or yoga class.
4. They can decide who will support them during labor and birth.
5. They may decide to use a doula.
6. They will pick a home birth, a birthing center birth, or a hospital birth!"

Alex put his head in his hands. "Too many decisions, Nonnie," he said. Tamika disagreed. "I like decisions. Nonnie, I heard my mom say you're often a doula for teen parents."

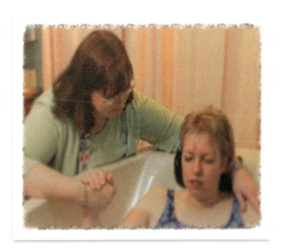
Nonnie's Doula Friend Ann

"I am," Nonnie said. "A doula is a person trained to support someone during labor and birth. It's an honor to be a doula."

Nonnie's Midwife Friend Venus

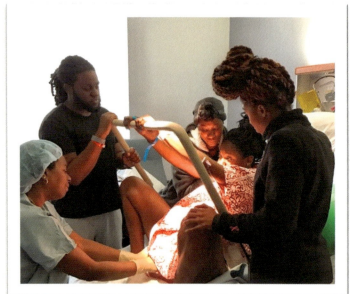

A midwife is a person who is trained to assist at birth. The midwife provides care during pregnancy and is present for labor and birth. Midwives are common in a lot of countries, including America.

An OB doc is an obstetrician—a specially trained doctor who also provides care during pregnancy, labor and birth. An obstetrician and a midwife may work together."

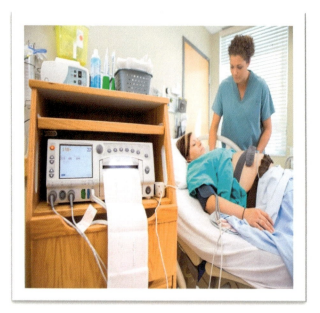

"What about where the baby is born?" Alex was very curious. "Why did my stepmom have Alisha at home?"

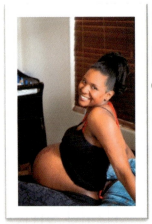

Nonnie shrugged. "Probably because her pregnancy was uncomplicated—meaning everything was going very well. Giving birth at home happened all the time years ago. Many people give birth at home today, because they like the idea of staying in a familiar place. Often, a midwife will attend a home birth."

The children stared at a picture in Nonnie's scrapbook.

"What's this?" Alex asked.

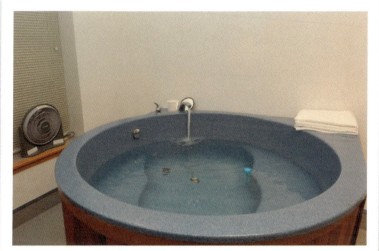

"It's a birthing pool. A person may choose a water birth. Giving birth in the water can happen at home or in a birthing center or hospital. The water can help during labor contractions."

"Giving birth in the water sounds wonderful." Tamika gushed.

"Wonderfully weird," said Alex. Tamika rolled her eyes at him, until he asked, "What's a labor contraction?"

"Labor is the word used to describe the process of birth. The uterus tightens and releases to help the birth happen. The tightening is called a contraction. Labor takes time."

"What do the contractions do?" Tamika asked.

"Contractions are the work of labor. Remember, the uterus is a muscle. It contracts—tightens—and releases over and over, until the uterus is ready for birth."

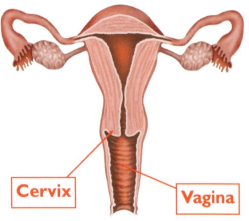

"The cervix—the bottom of the uterus—thins and opens during labor. The name for the opening is called dilatation. The cervix will dilate (open) to 10 cm so the baby can be born. After dilatation, the baby is pushed through the vagina. The vagina stretches. It is also called the birth canal."

"For a baby?" Alex asked, trying to picture it. He and Tamika exchanged looks. "Stretches for an entire baby?" Tamika asked.

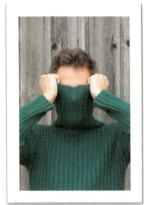

"Yes," Nonnie said, smiling. "The body knows what to do. Think of how a turtle neck sweater is pulled over someone's head. The baby comes through the birth canal like a sweater going over a head."

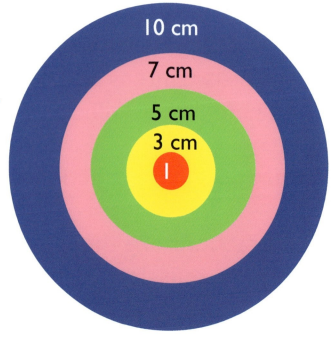

The cervix opens to 10 centimeters (CM).

The children were suddenly quiet.

Then they both said, "Wow!" and "Yippee" together, which made everyone laugh.

Nonnie showed another way to look at the cervix opening:

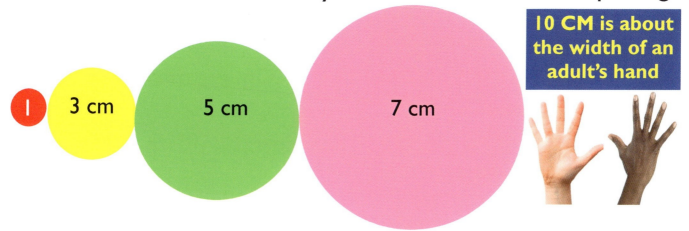

"Each birth is different," Nonnie continued. Check out this chart one of our young people created. It shows how labor contractions change and how the cervix opens."

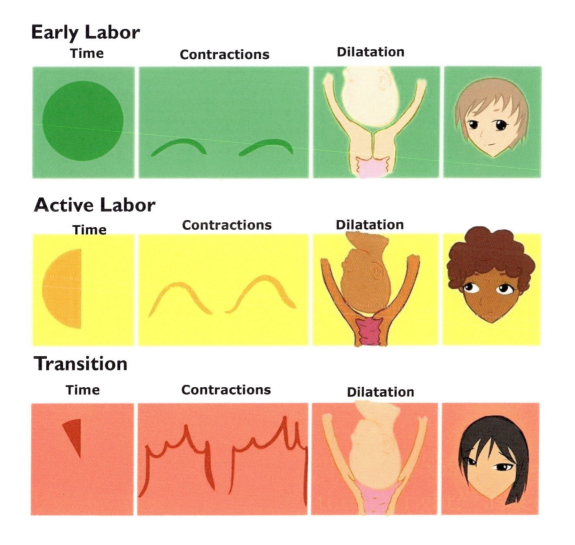

"When the cervix has thinned 100%—the fancy, medical word for thinning is effacement—and opened, or dilated to 10 cm, pushing can begin." Nonnie watched the children's expressions carefully. Were they still interested?

To her delight, they were not only interested, they had an important question!

"Does it hurt?" Tamika asked. "I think it would," added Alex, suddenly pleased he had no uterus.

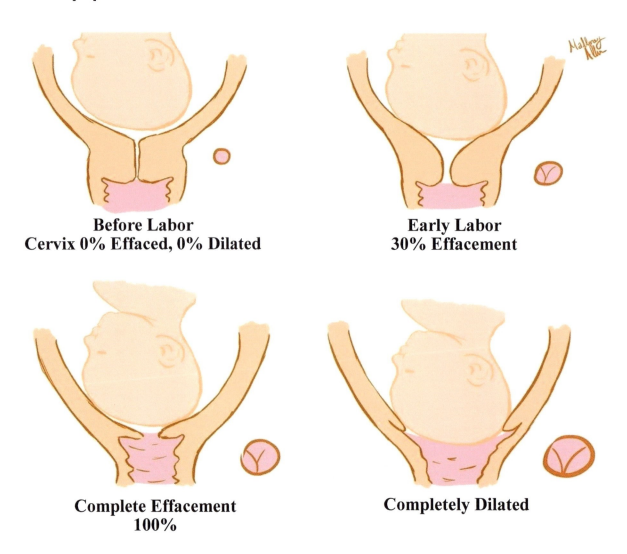

Before Labor
Cervix 0% Effaced, 0% Dilated

Early Labor
30% Effacement

Complete Effacement
100%

Completely Dilated

Nonnie thought their questions were outstanding.

"Pain is a very real part of life," she said. "Have either of you felt pain?"

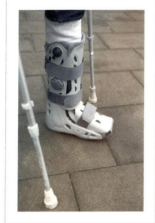

Tamika answered quickly. "Remember when I fell, Alex, and fractured my ankle? Yep. A broken ankle hurts!"

"I remember," Alex said. "It was hot and your skin was itchy."

Tamika grinned. "You helped carry my stuff at school."

"How about you, Alex?" Nonnie asked gently.

"Sure," Alex said. "When I had earaches all the time. I had tubes put in my ears. I was little, but I remember."

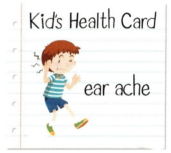

"Pain is scary," Nonnie said, "and usually tells us our bodies need help. Pain means something is wrong, or some part of us needs attention. The pain of labor is different. It's pain with a purpose."

"The purpose is the baby," Tamika said, beginning to understand.

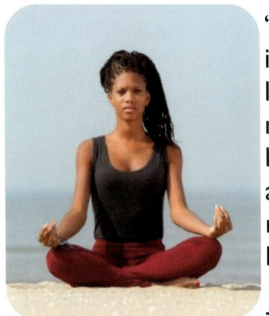

"Yes, Tamika. Preparing for birth includes learning about pregnancy, labor and birth," Nonnie said. "It means becoming aware of how the body gives birth. I teach relaxation and breathing to ease pain, and movement during labor to help the baby be born."

The children were very interested. Nonnie asked, "Would you like to try a little relaxation?"

They agreed. Nonnie said, "It's really easy. Your body belongs to you, so you can ease tension or feelings of stress whenever you wish. Please listen to my voice."

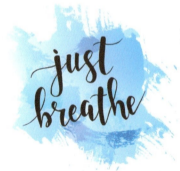

She told Tamika and Alex to do these things:
1. Close their eyes.
2. Think about a place where they felt very safe and happy.
3. Take a big breath in through their noses.
4. Think about breathing in.
5. Let the breath out through their mouths.
6. Think about breathing out.
7. Keep breathing, as slowly as they liked, over and over.
8. When they decide to stop, they should take a big breath, called a cleansing breath.

When they finished, Tamika said, "Your voice is so soft, Nonnie. I need you with me in school when I'm getting ready to take a test!"

"Thanks, Tamika," Nonnie grinned. "All you need is you. You can relax anywhere, all by yourself."

Birthing Ball
Movement can help with contractions. Using a birthing ball can ease pain.

She opened her scrapbook. "Check out these pictures of laboring mothers and their supportive partners.

A mother needs to know she is not alone. She needs someone to support her in labor."

Alex said, "I think being a doula would be a great job."

"It is," Nonnie said.

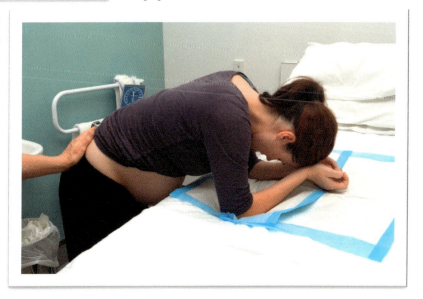

Labor support person applying back pressure to ease pain

The children were anxious to see more pictures.

Alex said, "Can we see how the baby comes out now? I'm ready."

"So am I," said Tamika excitedly.

Nonnie was pleased. "These are 3D pictures showing birth. Let's look at them, one at a time."

The children immediately had questions!

"Why is the baby all scrunched up?" Alex asked.

"There's not a lot of room in the uterus near the end of a pregnancy," Nonnie laughed.

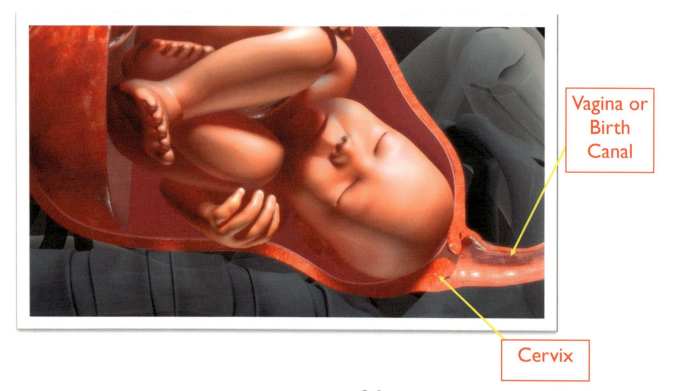

"Is the baby's head supposed to be down? It looks weird." Tamika frowned. "I think I'm glad I don't remember being born!"

Nonnie smiled. "Yes, honey. The head is the biggest part of the body. The baby needs to go through the pelvis, so it's nice to have the head go through first.

A female pelvis looks like this:

Female Pelvis

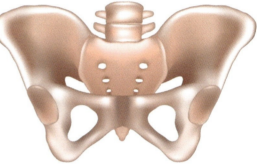

The baby fits inside the pelvis like this:

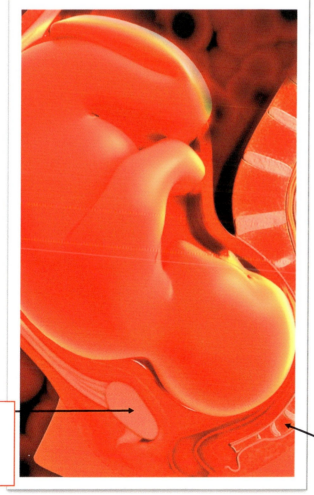

Front Pelvic Bone

Back Pelvic Bone

Can you see the way the baby is cradled by the pelvis before birth?

At the end of a pregnancy, most babies turn inside the uterus so their heads are down."

"Do you see how the cervix has thinned and opened?" Nonnie asked.

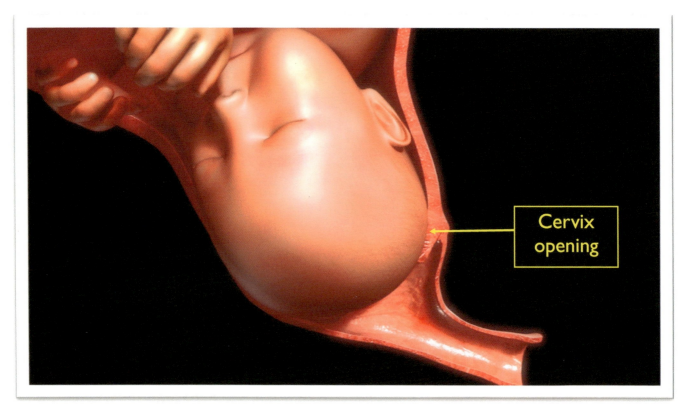

The children said, yes, then Alex said, "What happens next?"

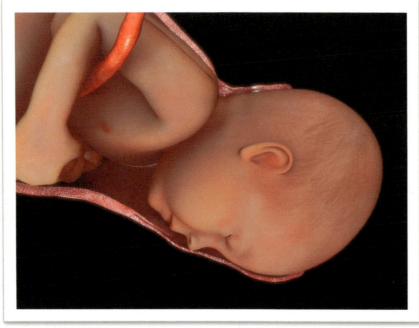

"The head begins to come down the vagina," Nonnie said. "This picture only shows the baby, not the rest of the mother's body. What do you notice about the head?"

"It's getting pointy," Alex stared at the picture.
"Like a conehead," added Tamika.

"Good observations," Nonnie said. "The head will adjust during birth so it fits well through the pelvis. A baby's skull has small places where the bone hasn't hardened, to allow the skull to move slightly. They're called fontanelles, or soft spots. After birth, the fontanelles will close over a period of time."

Fontanelles

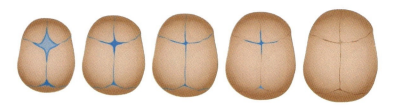

"Weird," said Alex. "Next, please," said Tamika.

"This picture," Nonnie explained, "shows a 3D representation of the baby starting to be born. You can see the midwife or doctor's hands. It's easiest if the mother is upright during this part of the birth."

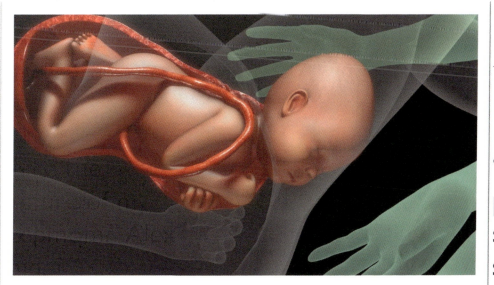

"Like the picture of my stepmom," Alex said.

"Yes, Alex," Nonnie said. "Just like when your stepmom gave birth to Alisha." She showed the children two more pictures from her scrapbook. The first was another 3D image.

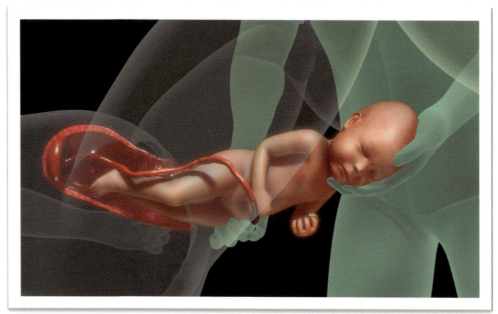

"Oh, wow, the baby is coming out!" Tamika laughed. "I know the picture isn't real, but it's cool."

"It is cool," Nonnie said. "Here's a picture of a real birth. My midwife friend Venus gave it to me. Can you see the baby's head? The father is helping the baby's birth."

"Double wow!" exclaimed Alex.

"Sweet!" said Tamika

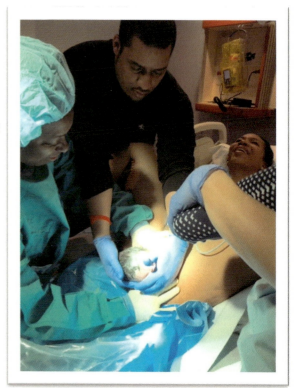

"If I'm ever a dad, I'll be at my baby's birth," Alex said.

Nonnie smiled. "I can't count how many births I've seen. I always feel so happy. Birth is an important part of life"

"What's a newborn look like?" Alex said. "I heard they look gross."

Nonnie said. "Babies can be slimy looking, but they're still great."

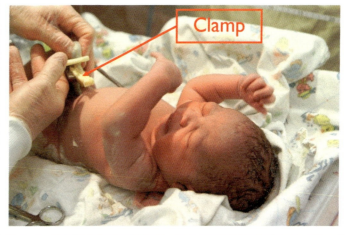

"What's that yellow thing?" Tamika pointed to the baby's belly.

Nonnie said. "It's a clamp used when the umbilical cord is cut." She hurriedly added, "Cutting the cord doesn't hurt the mother or the baby."

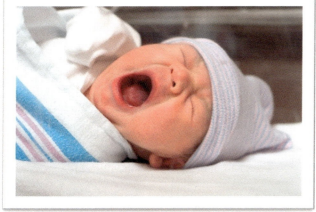

"What a sleepy baby," Alex said, smiling and looking at the book. "Being born must be tiring."

"Now I really can't wait to be a cousin!" Tamika said.

"Me too!" said Alex. "Wait a minute." Alex looked troubled. "Our friend RJ's mom just gave birth to his little sister, but she had an operation."

"A baby may be born through surgery. The abdomen and uterus are cut and the baby is removed. It's a cesarean birth." She flipped through the scrapbook for a picture. "The people dressed in blue are doctors and nurses."

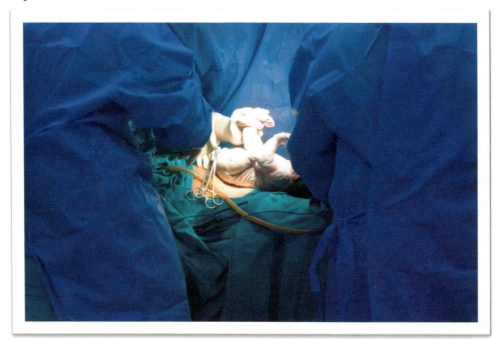

"Wouldn't that hurt the parent too much?" Tamika gasped.

"The parent is given anesthesia, usually an epidural, so the surgery isn't felt. An epidural can also be given during labor if wanted."

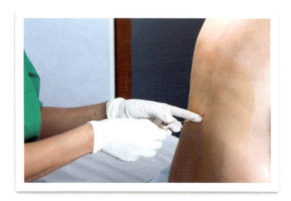

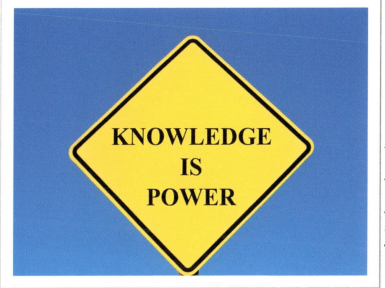

"I like knowing the truth about pregnancy and birth," Tamika said. "Remember when we talked giving birth in the water?" she asked. "Do you have any pictures of a water birth?"

Alex looked interested. "I'd like to see a picture of a water birth," he said.

"This baby is only minutes old," said Nonnie.

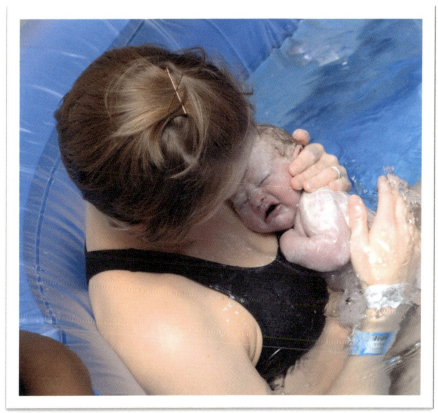

"Why does the baby's skin look like it's covered with lotion?" Alex asked. He was curious.

"Remember a baby is surrounded by amniotic fluid throughout pregnancy," Nonnie smiled. "It's amazing. The white cream on the baby's skin is called vernix. It covers and protects the baby."

"Wait a minute," Tamika said. "Time out. We talked about the placenta. Do you have a picture of it?"

"What's wrong with you, Tamika?" Alex teased. "This is gonna be gross."

"Some people think so," Nonnie said, suddenly serious. "Some things in life may seem gross, but they're still very important. The placenta keeps a new life alive for nine months!"

"I know," Alex said. "You're a nurse, though, Nonnie. Nothing is gross to you." Nonnie smiled, realizing her grandson was correct. She wasn't worried about body stuff. "It's just life, honey. Here's a picture of a placenta. You don't need to look at it."

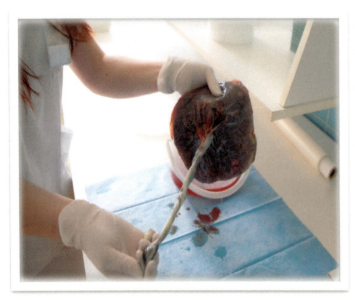

Alex sighed. "We've come this far," he said. Both children stared at the picture.

"Ewww," Tamika said. "Yuck," said Alex. Nonnie said, "Life can be yucky. I'm glad you're being honest."

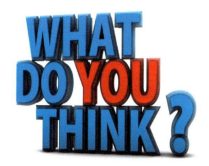

What do YOU Think?

Nonnie thinks birth is amazing.

Do you think giving birth is amazing?
Do you think it's gross?
Was there any part of birth that seemed strange?
What are your thoughts about birth?

Please draw or write your thoughts here:

Chapter Ten: Becoming a Family

"Will your Aunt Tracy breastfeed her baby?" Tamika asked Alex. "I know my mom nursed me. Breastmilk is good for babies."

Alex snorted, "How would I know?"

Tamika put her hands on her hips. "Listen here, Alex. Breastfeeding is perfect for babies. Stop thinking about breasts like they're just sexual."

Alex turned miserably to Nonnie, "I didn't. I don't. What did I say?"

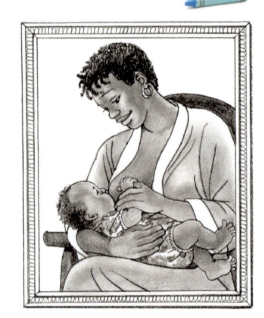

Nonnie said, "It's OK, both of you. You both know breastfeeding is normal. Tamika," she said calmly. "I actually have a picture of your mom nursing you when you were a baby."

"Wow," said Tamika.
"Not even yucky," said Alex, grinning.

"Sorry, Alex," Tamika said.

"You were a cute baby, Tamika," he said. Tamika gave him a huge hug.

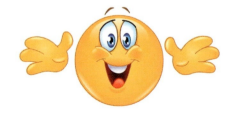

The children went home.

They went to school.

They waited. They waited some more!

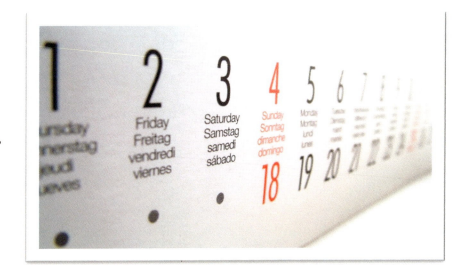

Finally, after days and days and weeks and weeks, they both were told the babies were born.

Tamika's Aunt Janell and Uncle David's baby was born first.

Both children couldn't wait to see the baby.

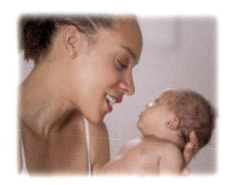

His name is Zion. He looks at his mom!

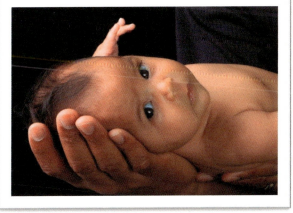

Zion fits in Uncle David's hands!

Tamika and Alex loved meeting little Zion.

"You're a cousin, Tamika," Alex said. "Yippee!"

Now, they needed to wait for Aunt Tracy's baby!

A week later, Alex's Aunt Tracy had her baby. Her birth was different. The placenta was low in the uterus, near the opening of the cervix. This is called placenta previa.

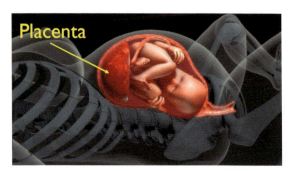

Typically the placenta is high inside the uterus. The midwife and doctor decided a cesarean birth would be safer. The parents agreed.

Aunt Tracy was prepared for a cesarean birth and her daughter was born!

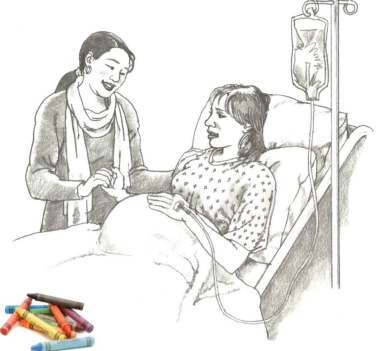

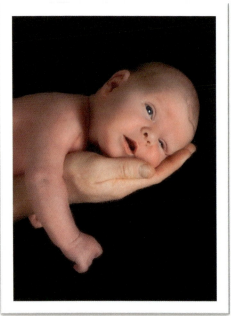

Her name is Lily. She has tiny feet!

Alex and Tamika loved meeting little Lily.

Lily fits in Uncle Ethan's hands!

"You're a cousin, Alex," Tamika cried. "Yippee!"

Families! Two new babies in two wonderful families!

Alex and Tamika are so happy.

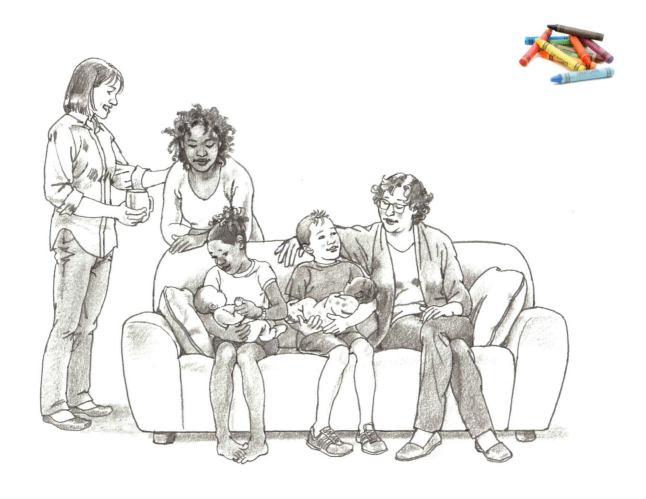

Tamika held Lily. Alex held Zion.
Nonnie came to visit.

When Nonnie saw Tamika and Alex and the beautiful babies, what do you think she said? If you guessed 'yippee', you are correct! What one word would you use to describe the feeling of having a new baby in a family?

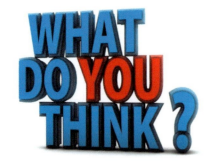

What do YOU Think?

Wow! Pregnancy and birth are very interesting!

Do you have any questions about pregnancy and birth? How do you feel about putting the puzzle together and learning about pregnancy and birth?

Please draw or write your thoughts here:

Glossary

10 cm (centimeters): how far the cervix of the uterus opens (dilates) before a baby can be born.

1st Trimester: The first part of a pregnancy, from week 1 to week 12.

2nd Trimester: The second part of a pregnancy, from week 13 to week 28.

3rd Trimester: The second part of a pregnancy, from week 49 to week 42.

Abdomen: The part of the body containing the stomach, intestines, liver and other organs; the belly.

Amniotic Fluid: Special liquid surrounding the fetus. The amniotic fluid is produced by a membrane surrounding the baby called the amnion. The fluid protects acts like a shock absorber and protects the growing fetus.

Anesthesia: Loss of feeling in a person's body; in surgery, due to drugs.

Anus: The opening of the GI (gastrointestinal) tract through which solid waste (stool or poop) leaves the body.

Belly Button: The place on the body where the umbilical cord is attached during pregnancy.

Birth Canal: Another name for vagina.

Birthing Ball: A large, rubber, air-filled ball that can be used for exercise or for a person in labor.

Birthing Center: A homey place where babies are born; it may be connected to a hospital..

Bladder: The organ where urine is stored.

Blastocyst: A structure formed in the early stages of a mammal's development. It has an inner cell mass which will form the embryo.

Breastfeed: To feed a baby human milk from milk ducts in the breast.

Cervix: The narrow, neck-like ending of the uterus—enters the vagina.

Cesarean Birth: When a baby is born through a surgical incision in the abdomen and uterus.

Glossary

Cleansing Breath: In mindful relaxation, one name for a big breath taken to center a person.

Contagious: Catchy. In the story, one of the children laughs because the other child is laughing.

Cousin: The child of a person's aunt or uncle.

Craving: Feeling like you want something, like a special food.

Differences : Things that make a person different or unique from other people.

Digestion: The process of taking nutrients from food to nurture the body; waste products are also removed.

Dilatation/Dilate: Open. In labor and birth, the cervix opens to 10 cm.

Doula: A person trained to support another person during labor and birth; a doula may also provide support after a baby is born.

Eaves-dropping: Listening secretly.

OB/Obstetrician: A medical doctor with special training to assist at labor and birth.

Effacement: Thinning. In labor and birth, the cervix thins 100%.

Egg: Also called an ovum, half of what is needed for fertilization.

Embryo: A developing unborn mammal. In humans, from the 2nd to the 8th week after fertilization, after which the name is fetus.

Engineer: A person who designs, builds, or maintains machines, buildings or public works.

Epidural: A type of anesthesia which causes a loss of feeling, usually below the waist.

Fallopian Tubes: A pair of tubes along which the egg travels from the ovary to the uterus.

Family Practice: A medical specialty including all aspects of family care.

Family Tree: A way of graphically explaining a family's background.

Glossary

Fertile: Able to reproduce.

Fertilization: When a sperm and egg unite.

Fetus: The name for an unborn mammal, especially a human, after the 8th week from fertilization.

Fontanelles: Spaces between the skull bones of a fetus or baby, where the sutures are not yet formed.

Half-sister: A sister with whom a sibling shares one parent.

Hormones: A natural chemical produced by the body that influences the way the body develops and grows.

Implants: In pregnancy, when a blastocyst adheres (sticks) to the uterine wall.

In Vitro Fertilization: A medical procedure whereby an egg is fertilized by a sperm in a test tube or outside the body.

Intrauterine Development: Growth after fertilization, inside the uterus.

Involuntary: In this case, a muscle the person does not control, like the uterus.

IUI: Intrauterine insemination—a type of fertility treatment where sperm are placed inside the uterus.

Labor: The birth process leading to the birth of the baby, the placenta, and the umbilical cord.

Labor Contractions: When the uterus tightens and releases to thin and dilate the cervix and allow the second stage (pushing) of labor to happen, leading to birth.

Lamaze®: A method of childbirth preparation promoting normal, natural birth through relaxation and breathing. Lamaze certified childbirth educators (LCCEs) are certified through Lamaze International.

Midwife: A person trained to assist a laboring person during childbirth. Midwives also provide pre-natal (before the birth) and post-partum (after the birth) care.

Miscarriage: The expulsion of a fetus from the uterus before it is able to survive independently.

Glossary

Muscle: Part of the body that has the ability to contract.

Myth: Something people believe that is not a fact.

Nausea: Feeling sick, feeling like throwing up.

Normalcy: When something is usual, typical, or common.

Nursing: In this case, another word for breastfeeding a baby.

Nutrients: A substance that provides nourishment to sustain life.

Ova: More than one egg. An ovum is one egg.

Ovary: The female body part where ova or eggs are produced.

Oxygen: A colorless, odorless gas that is necessary to sustain life.

Placenta: A temporary organ that joins the pregnant person and the fetus.

Placenta Previa: When the placenta is placed low in the uterus, blocking the baby's birth.

Placenta: Provides all nutrients and oxygen to the fetus.

Prenatal Exercise: Exercise done during pregnancy.

Prenatal Yoga: Special yoga classes and positions for pregnant.

Puberty: Growing from a child to an adult physical and emotionally.

Pubic Bone: Front bone of the pelvis (the bony cradle supporting the pregnant uterus).

Purpose: A reason something is done.

Rectum: The final section of the large intestine ending in the anus.

Relaxation: Being free from tension and anxiety.

Reproduction: The process of making a copy of something.

Sexual: Connected or related to sexuality.

Similarities: When something is the same.

Glossary

Sperm: One half of the cells needed for fertilization.

Spinal Column: Part of the spine that supports the body.

Toxoplasmosis: An infection caused by a parasite that is found in soil or cat feces (waste) that is harmful to a fetus.

Ultrasound: A scan of the uterus to visualize the fetus.

Umbilical Cord: Connects the fetus to the placenta; delivers oxygen and nutrients to the fetus. Removes waste from the fetus.

Uncomplicated: Easy, expected, smoothly done.

Uterus: Also called the "womb" - the muscle that houses the fetus.

Vagina: Tube from the uterus to the outside of a person's body.

Vaginal Opening: The opening to the vagina.

Veterinarian: A person trained to treat ill or hurt animals.

Vulva: The outside female body parts; the external genitals (genitals is a fancy name for those outside parts). Many people incorrectly use the term vagina for the vulva.

Zygote: A fertilized ovum.

Endorsements

Our children have so many important questions about the big topics in life. As a parent, it is a challenge to know what they can handle and how much to say. We always wish there was a guide to help us. Nonnie's newest book on pregnancy and birth gives us a structure to the conversation! Its respectful and honest tone invites discussion between adults and children who are reading it together. The illustrations give great visual context for the story and I am certain they will delight all. Sit down with your children and a favorite snack and let Nonnie lead the way!

~ Ann Grauer, AdvCD (DONA), Doula Coordinator at
Columbia Center Birth Hospital in Mequon, Wisconsin

Who else but Nonnie would reveal to children the secret that 'pregnancy means knowing how to find bathrooms'? Dr. Mary Jo Podgurski trusts children to find their way to understanding, provided they get the facts. 'Too many decisions, Nonnie,' says her main character, shaking his head—and we get the sense that his regard for those who carry and bear children, and those who support them to do so safely, has grown. Nonnie embodies this respect and makes it easy for her young audience to follow suit. Dr. Podgurski consistently sets a new standard of love and openness in all things.

~Anastasia Higginbotham, Author and illustrator of the Ordinary Terrible Things
children's series, published by the Feminist Press

It is so apparent that Nonnie, the author, knows her audience and how they learn. *Nonnie Talks About Pregnancy and Birth,* is a lesson for parents and children in so many more ways than just birth. Generations have left these topics undiscussed. Children don't know if it is okay to ask these questions and parents don't know how to discuss them with their children. This unique humanistic talk between a grandmother, her granddaughter and her granddaughter's friend gives us all lessons for respectful conversation about difficult topics. It is a gem for present and future generations.

~ Barbara A Hotelling, MSN, BSN, LCCE, IBCLC, WHNP
Duke University School of Nursing - Clinical Nurse Educator

This is a welcome addition to the "Nonnie" book series. Birth is an enormously important part of life, and one in which children of all ages are both curious and a bit afraid. Nonnie brings the children in, answering their questions, fully and honestly, cooking for them in between! The thoughtful teaching guided by the children's curiosity and questions bring the readers, and other children, into the conversation. Dr. Podgurski has an amazing ability to share her considerable knowledge and wisdom in simple ways that children can understand.

~ Judith Lothian, PhD, RN, LCCE, FAAN
Emeritus Director, Lamaze International Board of Directors

Nonnie Talks about Pregnancy and Birth is the book that I wish I had when I was a young girl. The words and images are informative but easy to understand. The language is accurate but not too wordy. Pregnancy can be a difficult and challenging subject to discuss with young people; however, Dr. Podgurski discusses both pregnancy and birth with sensitivity and insight. I'm looking forward to sharing this book with our 10 year old daughter. Thank you, Dr. Podgurski.

~ Ngozi D. Tibbs MPH, LCCE, IBCLC

Endorsements

Another great piece of work in the Nonnie series! This book about pregnancy and birth will stimulate open and honest conversations between parents or an trusted adult and young children.

~ Tara Owens Shuler, M.Ed., LCCE, FACCE, CD(DONA),
Lamaze Certified Childbirth Educator & Certified DONA Birth Doula

Dr. Mary Jo Podgurski --- one of the nation's most respected experts on pregnancy and childbirth --- has hit a homerun with the newest installment of the *Nonnie* series, *Nonnie Talks about Pregnancy and Birth*. "Nonnie" --- as warm, approachable, and deeply caring as the real-life version --- serves as a role model for answering children's questions in honest, respectful, and highly informative ways. Children will love the engaging illustrations as they relate to the storyline. Parents and other adult caregivers will trust that their children are receiving age-appropriate information. So choose your best comfy chair with the child you love, and welcome Nonnie to the family!

~ Bill Taverner, MA, CSE, Executive Director of The Center for Sex Education

Nonnie Talks About Pregnancy and Birth checks off all of the must-haves for a children's book about birth: truth, fun, respect, honesty, age appropriateness, and much more. Dr. Podgurski's conversational flow of interesting content will be eagerly received by children and their trusted grown-ups. If every child had a "Nonnie" in their life, how lucky and well-informed they would be!

~ Allison Walsh IBCLC, LCCE, FACCE

Nonnie Talks about Pregnancy and Birth is a must have for every parent's or school's bookshelf. In her unassuming and straightforward way, Dr. Mary Jo Podgurski walks young readers and their families through the story of pregnancy and birth with respect, knowledge, and an understanding that there are many different paths to becoming a family. Birth has long been a taboo subject because parents often lacked the tools with which to help them guide the discussion, this book is that long missing tool.

~ Robin Elise Weiss, PhD, AdvCD(DONA), CLC, LCCE, FACCE

What about those letters after people's names?

I can almost hear Tamika and Alex asking such a question!

The letters signify certifications; each letter reflects hours of work, experience, and dedication to excellence in a field of study.
I am proud to acknowledge my right to add these letters to my name:
LCCE (Lamaze Certified Childbirth Educator)
FACCE (Fellow in the American College of Childbirth Educators)
CSE (Certified Sexuality Educator)

Please encourage the young people in your life to reach for excellence!

Dr. Mary Jo Podgurski is the founder and director of The Washington Health System Teen Outreach and the Academy for Adolescent Health in Washington, Pa.

She is a nurse, a counselor, a parent, a trainer and speaker, and an educator who is dedicated to serving young people. The Outreach has reached over 230,000 young people since 1988. Check out www.healthyteens.com for information on the Academy and its programs.

Dr. Podgurski is certified as a childbirth educator through Lamaze International, (LCCE, FACCE) as a sexuality educator and a sexuality counselor through AASECT, as an Olweus Bullying Prevention Program trainer and through Parents As Teachers.

She is an authorized facilitator for the Darkness to Light abuse prevention program. Mary Jo is the author of the *Ask Mary Jo* weekly column in the Observer-Reporter newspaper and answers 6—10 questions from young people daily. She wrote Nonnie Talks about Gender as a labor of love and the Nonnie Series was birthed!

Most important, Mary Jo and her partner Rich are the parents of three wonderful adult children and are blessed to be grandparents. She is a Nonnie in Real Life!

Dr. Podgurski believes ally is a verb.
She believes in social and racial justice.
She believes in young people.
She believes each person is a person of worth. Please pass it on.

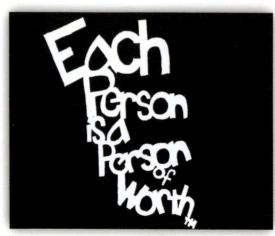

ABOUT THE NONNIE SERIES

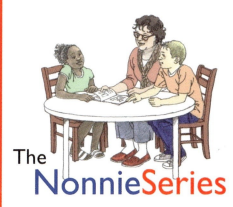

Writing Nonnie Talks about Gender in the summer of 2014 was a true labor of love. The idea of a "Nonnie Series" never entered my mind.

The reactions I've had to Nonnie Talks about Gender surprised and humbled me. I began to realize gender wasn't the only challenging topic in our world. Social media and 24 hour news have created information overload, where even elementary school children are inundated with potentially confusing and troubling subjects. How should adults open the door to these teachable moments?

As a young nurse I became a birth advocate; as a certified Lamaze childbirth educator I have continued my commitment to birthing women and families since the 70s. In 1973, I began working with pediatric oncology at Memorial Sloan Kettering Cancer Center in New York City. My passion for birthing normally dovetailed with my growing commitment for death with dignity. I became a hospice nurse in the 80s. Long before the "circle of life" became part of a popular film for children, I learned how vital birth and death are to the human experience...and how often both topics are avoided when talking with children.

With birth and death advocacy as my foundation, I decided to tackle these subjects in books for children as part of a series based on the "Nonnie" concept. I started storyboards on both topics. Then, life intervened.

As an ally and advocate for racial and social justice, I cannot ignore how much our culture needs to address racial equity. Then, as I was presenting my child abuse prevention program, *Inside Out, Your Body is Amazing Inside and Out and Belongs Only to YOU*, an eight year old child told me what #BlackLivesMatter meant to her. We talked, I listened. This little one's very real fear that her own life was less worthy than another's based on the color of her skin was my inspiration for Nonnie Talks about Race.

Nonnie Talks about Puberty was born because another child needed it. I began teaching growing up classes called What's Up as You Grow Up in 1984. Gender non-conforming children are often confused during puberty; I couldn't find an inclusive resource on growing up, so I wrote one. Empathy is a learned skill. I hope all children will benefit from the information in Nonnie Talks about Puberty.

Nonnie Talks about Pregnancy and Birth is a natural result of a life spent as a birth advocate. I now plan to write Nonnie Talks about Death and Nonnie Talks about Mental Health. I have a list of other topics I hope to address. If you have any ideas for the Nonnie Series, or would like to be informed about coming titles, please connect with me at podmj@healthyteens.com.

Did you enjoy Nonnie Talks about Pregnancy and Birth?
Interested in Nonnie Talks about Puberty?
Curious about Nonnie Talks about Race?
Intrigued by Nonnie Talks about Gender?
Entranced by the concept of the Nonnie Series?

Dr. Podgurski has dedicated her life to empowering young people.
She strives to model her motto of "Each Person is a Person of Worth"
through education, writing, and trainings.
She is available for workshops and consultation.
She is also the author of 26 books.
You can find her books, including the Nonnie Series, at Amazon or
on her website, www.healthyteens.com
You can reach her at:

Email: podmj@healthyteens.con
Toll free #: 1 (888) 301-2311
Twitter DrMaryJoPod

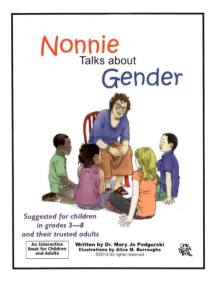

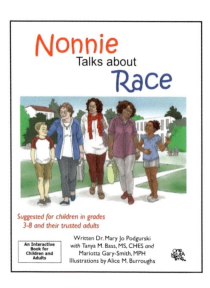

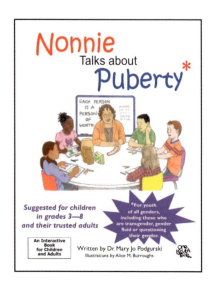

Printed in Great Britain
by Amazon